Peaceful Breeze

Mark Carrington

Clink Street

London | New York

Published by Clink Street Publishing 2017

ISBN: 978-1-911110-30-9 paperback
978-1-911110-31-6 ebook

In Memory of Marian Rose Carrington (1935-2015)
By her son Mark

Sometimes life goes the way you want
And sometimes it doesn't
And when it doesn't, if you look,
you will find something beautiful
Anonymous Quote

Contents

About the author

I have always been a goal-oriented person. Achieving just about anything I really set my mind to. This includes securing three master's degrees over my life.

Then in early 2014, my entire world turned upside down. My mother was diagnosed with advanced colon cancer. She passed away in June 2015.

Through the daily challenges of caring and nursing for Mum, I discovered a wellspring of inner strength that I never knew I possessed. As a result of my personal brokenness, paradoxically, today I am a much stronger person. The quote from the famous German philosopher Friedrich Nietzsche is so true. He said "That which does not kill us, makes us stronger." Not only have I discovered who I am. I now have a clearer sense of my purpose in this world.

Throughout her illness, I witnessed something truly wonderful, Mum's humanity. Caring for Mum has profoundly changed my life. I now know what it means to be human. I am even more determined to love and cherish my family and friends. Above all, I am going to try to live the best life I can. I am now planning to study towards a Doctorate of Philosophy (PhD) in Palliative Care. I have this insatiable desire within me, as long as I live, I will learn.

In my wildest imagination I could have never envisaged writing a book on this topic. In some small way, I hope my story will help other carers who are looking after a loved one with a terminal illness.

All the events and conversations contained in the book are true.

Introduction

Witnessing Mum's sheer vulnerability and the purity of her love as she succumbed to her cancer was a truly humbling and profound experience.

Everyone diagnosed with a terminal illness has a different story, a different experience, and a different way of approaching the end of their life.

For family members caring for those loved ones, it can be an equally traumatic time. They too have their story to tell.

This book chronicles my story, both as a son and as Mum's carer. In particular, as strange as it may sound, it gave me the opportunity to understand myself better and more importantly, grow as an individual.

In 2014, Mum was diagnosed with advanced colorectal cancer, also known as colon, bowel, or rectal cancer.

This book records our journey and experiences as we navigated through the healthcare sector. In particular, how doctors, nurses, and healthcare professionals treated Mum at every stage throughout her illness.

Overall, Mum was treated well as a cancer patient. As she neared the end of her life, however, the coordination, delivery and quality of the palliative care, was on occasions, sub-standard. Often, the lack of compassion and tenderness she received was woeful.

The harsh reality is that if you are frail, elderly, vulnerable, and seriously ill, you simply do not have the strength to complain or stand up against how you are being treated by the healthcare professionals. If it had not been for me standing beside her as her advocate throughout her illness, Mum would have suffered in silence, like many thousands of elderly people.

As Mum was a gentle woman, she did not want any fuss to be made over her. She did not wish to place a burden on anyone dealing with her illness, whether it be the doctors, nurses, or the care team looking after her. She repeatedly apologised to them for actually being ill. As you read through this book, you will see the emotional rollercoaster ride I went through and the tensions I had to face while constantly fighting on Mum's behalf to ensure she was given the best medical treatment and care possible.

In my opinion, at any point during Mum's diagnosis, she could have so easily fallen through the gaps in the healthcare system. She could have so easily died a premature, terrible, and tragic death. As it happened, she passed away with dignity in a hospice.

I hope this book serves as more than just a grief memoir, and instead encourages a wider debate about our society's view of caring for our loved ones when they are reaching the end of their life.

The need for both social and end-of-life care is going to rise exponentially. The biggest challenge for our society is how we look after the elderly in the context of fiscal and budgetary restraints within the National Health Service (NHS) against the backdrop of finite resources.

The facts are shocking. For example, you might be startled to know that:
- The population over 75 is projected to double in the next 30 years.
- There are over a million carers over 65, an increase of a quarter in the last ten years.
- Two-thirds of hospital patients are now over 65.

While we have a strong hospice movement, just over five percent of us will pass away in a hospice with world-class care. The reality is that the majority of us will pass away in a hospital.

The core principles of the NHS are focused on early detection, treatment, and survivorship of our illnesses. I strongly believe that palliative and end-of-life care must be included as a further core principle. Without it, many of us will continue to die without dignity.

With the advances in medicine and the longevity of life, the ethical choices of end-of-life care are not so simple.

The right to die discussion is not what this book is about. There are plenty of books that cover this subject area. The law in the UK as it stands is clear: assisting someone to die is illegal. The rights of the person to determine and exercise how and when they wish to die, and the counter-argument that such a decision essentially undermines religious, philosophical, and ethical principles, will continue to be debated by society for decades to come.

Who this book is for

I believe there is something very precious and life-transforming about caring for a loved one.

So, before I outline who this book is for, I need to tell you "who this book isn't for."

When you care for a loved one, you do things not out of a sense of duty, but out of pure selfless love.

If you are caring for someone you do not love or have no empathy for, then this book is probably not for you. You will not understand the heartache and, at times, the sheer indescribable joy of caring for a loved one.

No one who hasn't been the primary carer of someone with a chronic or terminal illness for an extended period can begin to imagine what it is like. You can read book after book about caring for a loved one. But it is only when it happens to you that you truly understand the impact it has on your life.

For me, caring for Mum was like second nature, as natural as breathing.

It was that unconditional love that sustained me through the difficult and unexpected journey we faced.

I trust that this book, somehow, gives you an idea of what it is like.

If you are caring for a loved one, I hope this book will provide comfort and reassurance that you are not alone. Millions of other people, including myself, have trodden this path before you.

Why I wrote this book

I have thought long and hard about writing about my experience of caring for Mum. It has been an incredibly hard decision to make. But in the end, I boiled it down to four reasons.

First, to honour my Mum, her memory, and her humanity.

Second, I hope this book will help other carers going through the same experience.

After reading this book, you will see how, as a carer, I navigated through the depths of unmanageable emotional pain as I accompanied Mum to the end of her life. I believe you cannot go through an experience of caring for a loved one with a terminal illness and remain unchanged as a person.

If even just one person going through the heartache of caring for a loved one with a terminal illness reads this book and it helps them, then that's enough for me; I'll have done my job.

And thirdly, through deep emotional writing I have been able to gain perspective over my loss, and to gain power over my grief.

Finally, I believe we should protect the vulnerable and preserve their dignity not only while they are living, but also as they reach the end of their life.

In this respect, the book is dedicated to the many thousands of carers who selflessly look after their terminally ill loved ones.

Key lessons

There are four key lessons that I have learnt caring for Mum, which I hope you can take away from reading this book.

First, I just simply kept on digging deeper into my emotional reserves. And when I thought I had reached the bottom, I managed, as a carer, to somehow dig deeper. And day after day, I continually dug deeper.

Believe me when I say you are emotionally stronger and more resilient than you think. You just need to know how to tap into your hidden strengths to pull you through. For me, it was my faith and the power of prayer.

I hope you will see, as you read about my personal journey as a carer, how I managed to draw on my emotional reserves.

The second key lesson is one of forgiveness. By which I mean forgiveness not only of others, but more importantly of myself. Let me explain. There were times when I was caring for Mum, I would become angry, frustrated, and annoyed. I might have said things to her in the wrong tone or in a raised voice. I now regret that. I have regrets for things I should have done differently or not done at all when caring for her.

I wish I could take back my anger and not have raised my voice or been consumed by my emotions. But I can't. There is no rewind button in life. The past cannot be undone. I made a lot of mistakes when caring for Mum. It has taken me over a year, to accept my own failings and weaknesses as her carer but more importantly as her son. I have found peace, in the knowledge, that as I was going through this heartrending period of my life, I followed my inner voice. In effect, my soul. I tried to do my best. I tried to do the right thing by Mum. And that is, in my opinion, all you can do in life. The third key lesson is one of letting go. No matter how much you love a person, ultimately, it is their personal journey. The hardest thing I had to do in my life was to let go of Mum. That is not to say I do not miss her every day, because I do. More than I can express in words. She is in my mind and heart every single day. I accepted, however, that it was her journey to take alone. Getting to that point of profound understanding, I first had to take a journey of self-discovery. It did not happen instantly or overnight. It is only now, looking back, that I realised, running in parallel with Mum's journey, I too was on my own journey of self-realization.

Finally, and not least, is the use of humour. It is strange to say, but there were moments of pure joy for caring for mum. I believe in the right circumstances and in the right context, humour can ease emotional pain.

When you care for someone you love, it deepens your empathy, your compassion, and your humanity. For me, to witness the sheer frailty of my Mum, another human being, has transformed my own life in so many ways I thought were not possible.

About mum

This book is primarily about my emotional journey of caring for my mother.

I do, however, wish to give you a brief insight into the type of person Mum was. To describe her as a 'cardboard cut out of a saint', would not give her life justice. She was very much alive and wanted to live. The early part of her life can only be described as tough and unfair. The university of life was not kind to her. But she got through it. I have no doubt these years developed her indomitable spirit.

As an only child, I was my Mum's pride and joy. And like most mothers, even when I was a grown adult, she still saw me as her little son. Whenever life got tough for me, she was the one who kept me going and encouraged me not to give in.

Mum was loving, caring, and thought of others first. She was warm and open-hearted. She not only stood up for fairness and justice, but she would fight for the poor and the underprivileged in our society. She knew first-hand how tough life could be because when she was young, trying to put food on the table was a daily struggle. But she never let the poverty affect me.

She was also a woman with integrity, compassion, honour, respect, kindness, and love.

Mum enjoyed watching sports on television. In particular, horse racing and football. She was an avid and knowledgeable supporter of Arsenal Football Club. She could name all the great players: Thierry Henry, Dennis Bergkamp, Ian Wright, and Robin van Persie, to mention just a few.

Mum wasn't the type of person who could share her emotions and feelings easily.

She was a neat and organised person—everything had to have a place and a purpose. At times, this used to drive me crazy. But that was the way she was.

Mum was four years old when the Second World War began and ten when it ended.

As a child, she grew up in a world where bombs were being dropped only a few houses away from her. She loved to tell me her memories of when the family used to live on Homer Street in Paddington, London. She told me how, as a child, she crawled under the table when the bombs were being dropped. All the houses in the street had lost their roofs and windows. "We were very lucky," she commented as she reminisced.

She would also reminisce about how she was evacuated to Wolverhampton for a short period during the war with her niece Shirley, and how the couple that looked after them in Wolverhampton wanted to keep her. But my grandmother (Mum's mum) would never entertain such a thought. She always said my grandmother was a "golden mum."

Perhaps her childhood contained her fondest memories as she was surrounded with so much love. Whilst times were tough in those days, there was a shared community (where people looked out for each other), a shared purpose and spirit. She often told me about how she rode her first bike and how she cried watching the Disney film *Bambi*. She would often say to me that, whilst money was short and food was rationed, they were nevertheless, lovely years to live through. Listening to her memories were truly beautiful moments for me.

Mum continued throughout her life to have a war-like spirit of just getting on with life, no matter what she faced. That spirit has been instilled in me.

Mum was not particularly religious, but she retained a faith and spiritual belief that she kept to herself.

To Mum, being polite and having manners was part of her belief in living a good life.

As I was growing up, Mum gave me three pieces of advice.

The first was always to be grateful. She used to say, "There but for the grace of God go I."

Second, "Do unto others as you want them to do unto you." In other words, treat people as you wish to be treated.

And finally, she told me always to find a sanctuary inside myself, inside my heart, that no one is allowed to invade. "That space is yours alone, where you find your inner peace and contentment," she used to tell me. "Only you and you alone can make yourself happy."

Above all, as you read through this book, you will see that she was resilient to the very end.

She always maintained, as she got older, that the fear of death had faded into an acquiescence and recognition. She just hoped she would die peacefully. As a consequence, she not only accepted her terminal illness, but faced it head on with courage and fortitude. At no stage during her illness did she say she wanted to give in or give up. She had a fighting spirit and an insatiable will to live.

To me, she was, and will always remain, a simply remarkable woman who lived a worthy, simple, and contented life with gracefulness and purpose.

Surely, that is all we can hope for in our own lives.

1

The Journey Begins

Even though my lifestyle has been insulated and my life largely untested, I thought I had a sense of mastery and choice over my life. As a goal-oriented person, I had all my hopes and plans laid out in front of me and, one by one, I was achieving them. Whilst never being complacent, I lived in my own little world. I thought I was in control of my life and destiny.

Everything changed forever on a cold rainy day. It was Friday, 14th March 2014. As usual, I left home for work at 7:30 am. Mum went out to do her daily shopping. She always liked to buy fresh vegetables and fruit. She would walk at least two miles a day—a mile to the shops and a mile back. That was pretty good for a 79-year old woman.

But on this particular day, as Mum was walking down the high street, out of nowhere someone tripped her up.

Apparently, it was a young man running to catch a bus. Mum was walking in front of him at the time. The man tripped her from behind by clipping one of her heels. She fell down on the ground. Fortunately, she fell in such a way that she managed to avoid hitting her head. The young man failed to stop. He shouted, "Get out of my way, old woman, I'm late for work." He subsequently caught his bus. The incident was over in a split second.

Bystanders helped Mum up from the ground. She was visibly shaken. "I just want to go home and have a cup of tea," she said politely. She thanked all the people who helped her. She brushed her coat down and, without any assistance, walked home by herself.

I was at work during the time of the incident. When I phoned her during my lunch break, she reluctantly told me she had fallen. But she insisted there was nothing to worry about. I immediately rushed home and discovered she had bruises on her elbow and around her face. It was as if she had gone three rounds with the boxer Mike Tyson. She didn't want to go to the local hospital. In fact, she didn't want any fuss made over her.

Soon after the fall, I noticed Mum wasn't her usual self. She was anxious, fearful, and apprehensive. It was unlike her. She had suddenly lost her confidence. Since her fall, she would gaze out the kitchen window each evening, waiting for me to arrive home from work. She kept pleading for me to come home early.

On Tuesday, 1st April 2014, I suffered a bout of food poisoning. I laid in bed in agony. All I could remember is feeling sorry for myself.

At the exact moment I was delving deep into my own self-pity, Mum started to develop diarrhoea. We both naturally thought her diarrhoea was somehow connected to my food poisoning. That day, Mum asked me to go to the local pharmacy in order to buy some anti-diarrhoea medication. We both took the tablets, but whilst my diarrhoea stopped in a few days, Mum's continued. The tablets simply had no effect on her.

Mum's diarrhoea persisted for at least a week. Then, soon after, she started to feel constipated. I subsequently bought some constipation tablets from the pharmacy. They didn't work either. Mum was now in considerable discomfort. At this stage, we didn't know what to do. I then started to notice Mum was leaving her meals. She had never had a large appetite, but I could see she was not eating normally. I also subsequently discovered she was not eating during the day when I was at work.

I could see her symptoms becoming more acute since the fall. There was no doubt in my mind that Mum's fall was the event that triggered her sudden deterioration. Looking back, I am sure the fall was the catalyst for the cancer cells to accelerate their growth within her body.

I tried to explain to her that it would be a good idea to see a doctor. But she refused point blank to be medically examined. Day after day, I would beg her to go. But the more I kept on pleading with her, the more stubborn she would become. I simply could not get through to her.

"Stop fussing over me," she kept saying apologetically.

"I'm your son. I'm always going to fuss over you. I care," I repeatedly replied.

The situation deteriorated. We would often get into a stand-off situation. I would often become frustrated, exasperated, and annoyed with her. Sometimes, I would slightly raise my voice to her. Then at night, I would lie awake feeling guilty for having these emotions in me. Night after night I barely slept, thinking about how I could convince her to see the doctor. I just could not find the right vocabulary that would persuade her. I felt I was letting Mum down.

The next day, I arranged for the next-door neighbour to come round and see Mum. Even the neighbour couldn't persuade her. Mum wouldn't even listen to her brothers or sisters, who again pleaded with her to be examined by the doctor.

"I will go in my own time," she said. "You are worrying about nothing. We are just going to waste the doctor's time."

"Do you think I am going to leave you like this?" I exclaimed sympathetically.

The reality, of course, was that Mum was in denial. And there was nothing I could do about it.

Despite her refusal to see sense, I could see she was anxious, scared, and fearful of what the doctor might say. Deep down inside, she knew something was wrong with her body. Also, I believe she was genuinely embarrassed. She did not want to talk about medical matters below her waistline. Given her age and the generation she grew up in, in hindsight, I should have understood more about the level of her embarrassment and self-consciousness. I regret this now.

I made an appointment to see a private medical consultant in order to seek his professional opinion, as to whether I could force Mum to see a doctor. I did so without her knowledge. It was my final attempt to help her.

He advised me that unless I had the power of attorney, I could not force her to seek medical treatment. "It appears your mum is of sound mind," he concluded. "She is not incapable of making decisions. She is not suffering from dementia or Alzheimer's disease. Mark, there is nothing you can do. You just simply have to accept her decision." He solemnly concluded.

The next day, I could see that she was becoming more and more breathless. She could hardly manage to walk. Even getting up from the sofa into a standing position required every ounce of her strength. The turning point came one day, when she could not stand up from sitting on the sofa. She needed my assistance. I wrapped my arms underneath both her shoulders and then, with a gentle push, I lifted her up.

She then finally accepted that she was ill. That in itself was a blessing. In total, it took four weeks for Mum to go reluctantly to see the doctor.

I was so pleased and relieved that she had made the decision. Although I was reassured that she was finally in the healthcare system, I knew her journey had only just begun.

It was Friday, 2nd May 2014. The doctor's surgery was about a fifteen-minute walk from home. With Mum clinging to my arm, we arrived five minutes before her appointment. Mum grumbled and muttered repeatedly throughout our walk, "I don't want to go to see the doctor."

When we finally arrived, we had to queue to see the doctor's receptionist. It was going to be the first of many memorable and precious moments I can recall.

The receptionist asked Mum which doctor she wished to see.

"Doctor Coleman," Mum replied.

"We don't have a Doctor Coleman working here. When was the last time he saw you?" The receptionist politely asked.

"In 1981," Mum replied with a deadpan expression on her face.

The receptionist looked amazed. I started to grin discreetly, which then immediately turned into a smile.

In so many ways, Mum had been blessed because she had never really been ill for the vast majority of her life. She simply did not entertain going to the doctor for anything. She did not have any women's health screenings throughout her life. She would always say to me, "Your health is your wealth. I've never had money in life, but I've had my health."

Given what I know now, it is highly likely that the colon tumour had remained dormant and silent for many years inside her. Every cell in our body contains DNA. In Mum's case, the gene mutations of these cells, unbeknown to her, were building up slowly over decades.

Eventually the cancerous cells accumulated to such a mass, over a very short period of time, they started to eat away at her vital organs.

Without ever having been medically assessed, cancer could have cost her life at a much younger age. In this respect, Mum won the jackpot in life. Not in monetary terms, but with the span of her good health throughout her life.

Thankfully, the doctor saw Mum on that day. We waited about an hour in reception and then the doctor called out her name. She wanted to see the doctor alone. "I am here waiting for you," I said, continually reassuring her. I waited in reception as she shuffled into the doctor's room.

Within fifteen minutes, Mum came out. She sat down. "The doctor looked very serious. I think I have diabetes," she worryingly concluded.

The doctor immediately referred her for an urgent appointment for a combined colonoscopy and endoscopy followed by a consultation with the oncologist consultant at St John's Hospital.

"We just have to wait and see what they say at the hospital," I replied calmly, trying to reassure her. I knew, however, that her condition was far more serious.

Back home, we needed to make some quick decisions about our living arrangements.

At this stage, Mum could not handle the two flights of stairs to her bedroom or to the bathroom. She wanted to sleep on the sofa in the living room. Again, she didn't want any fuss made over her. In many respects, it made sense as we had, fortunately, a downstairs toilet she could use. We agreed she could have a daily wash in the kitchen. While Mum was feeling ill, she was still in no rush to have the combined colonoscopy and endoscopy procedure.

Fortunately, I had some annual leave owed to me at work, so I decided to take a month off work to look after Mum twenty-four hours a day. My employer at this stage could not be more helpful, which I thought was strange at the time, given they were not friendly towards me. I thought nothing of it and was grateful for the time off.

Two weeks after seeing the doctor, Mum received a letter from St John's Hospital, saying that she was due to have the procedure on Tuesday, 3rd June 2014. To say she wasn't looking forward to it would have been an understatement. Mum was more worried about the procedure itself rather than the outcome of the results from it.

On 2nd June 2014, the day before the procedure, she had to drink a laxative solution. She was supposed to have it twice during the day, once at noon and once at 6 pm. After I had made up her first solution, Mum drank it in one go. I told her not to drink it like that, but she wouldn't listen. About two minutes afterwards, she started to vomit violently. I didn't know what to do, so I immediately rang the out-of-hours service. The nurse on the phone advised Mum just to take tiny sips of the solution throughout the day.

After Mum followed her advice, the laxative started working. That day, Mum spent hours in the bathroom.

On the day of the procedure, we arrived early at the main reception. Mum was visibly anxious. Once she saw the doctor, however, who explained the procedure, she seemed to be more at ease. All the doctors and nurses were professional, well informed, and so very kind to her.

During the combined colonoscopy and endoscopy, the doctor put a small camera up Mum's back passage and down her throat. She was not given a general anaesthetic for the procedure. Instead they gave her a mild sedative.

About three hours later, the nurse contacted me and confirmed I could see her. As I walked into the ward, Mum was sitting up in her bed drinking a cup of tea. She looked so frail. "This is my angel," she announced proudly to the nurse while pointing to me. The nurse smiled.

Not wanting Mum to see the tears flowing down my face, I had to turn quickly away.

The nurse explained the medical procedure had gone well, but there were a few things that "looked worrying". She then advised me they were going to send for further tests to understand the abnormalities of some polyps. Mum stayed in the hospital for one night. As I left for home, the nurse pulled me to one side and said softly to me, "Mark, your Mum will be in safe hands. But it is important you should know that you need to hope for the best but plan for the worst." I looked at her with my eyes still watering with tears, thanked her, and acknowledged that I fully understood what she was saying.

Until that time, cancer had not been something we thought about on a daily basis. Due to my own foolishness, I never imagined colon cancer would strike someone I loved. My ignorance will haunt me until the day I die, as I should have looked out for the signs of Mum's deterioration.

Now, more than a year later, I repeatedly ask myself how I failed to add up the signs that Mum had colon cancer. But I honestly didn't see them. There weren't any flashing warning signals saying to me that this could have been cancer. Or if there were, they were not visible to me.

Of course, I noticed Mum was becoming frailer, slower, and her demeanor more vulnerable. If I am truly honest with myself, I did, however, notice some weight loss, especially in her face. But I simply put it down to old age. Never in a moment of my thoughts did I think she had cancer.

It had never occurred to Mum she would die of cancer. She had always thought she would die of heart failure. Cancer seemed to happen to other people, not to us. The terrible truth, however, was that it was happening to us right now, right this minute.

She was in total disbelief. She was scared, bewildered, confused, and angry. She had never smoked or drunk alcohol in her entire life. She had always eaten healthily. "How can this happen to me? It seems so unfair," she kept repeating. Whether it was unfair or not, we were suddenly being dragged into a direction in life not of our choosing. We were embarking on a journey into the unknown.

Mum did not fear death. But she was fearful of the process of dying. She feared going into the unknown. She feared the pain that cancer could cause. She feared humiliation and degradation. She was afraid of incontinence. And the loss of her independence. Ultimately, she feared losing her dignity.

Over the course of a month or so, cancer seemed to be everywhere I looked. It was ubiquitous. It pervaded my life.

I would turn on both the BBC and Sky news. At the time, a new report on cancer had just been published—one in three people is diagnosed with cancer. By 2030, the number of people living with cancer in the UK is predicted to double from two million to four million. Whenever I turned on the radio, there was talk about cancer.

I would pass a newspaper stand and all I could see were the front-page headlines of celebrity after celebrity passing away from cancer.

I would walk down the street and see massive billboards about cancer. Or when I was doing the shopping, cancer charities would stop me on the street asking for donations.

After the combined colonoscopy and endoscopy procedure, it was another three weeks before Mum saw the oncologist. Once again, she was in no rush to attend the appointment. The hospital even allowed us to move the appointment earlier, but Mum didn't want to cause any fuss to anyone. If she had her way, she would have been quite happy to postpone the appointment indefinitely.

In the meantime, Mum was rapidly deteriorating. She was becoming frailer and losing a significant amount of weight. She was increasingly more lethargic. She also looked jaundiced. She was now starting to get breathless, even when she was sitting down.

We were due to see the oncologist three days after my birthday, on Tuesday, 24th June 2014.

Typical of Mum, she was more worried about my birthday than herself and her illness. "For the first time in my life, I can't go out and buy you a birthday card," she said with a tear in her eye. So as a compromise, she gave me a few pounds from her weekly pension money so I could go out and buy a card from the shop.

2

The diagnosis

When you are caring for someone you love, there are certain key dates you will never forget. Listening to the diagnosis of a loved one saying that he or she has a terminal illness is one of them.

We arrived at the hospital early. Mum's appointment was at 11 am. We were told, however, that the oncologist was running late. So we had to wait a further two hours before we were finally led into his office.

Mr Carmichael greeted us. "Please do come in and take a seat," he advised in a self-assured and professional tone.

Straight away, Mr Carmichael could see Mum was anaemic and malnourished.

Five minutes afterwards, the nurse walked into the room.

After examining Mum on a medical bed in his room, Mr Carmichael sat down in his chair and started typing on his computer. He looked solemn. We were both sitting there, waiting in total apprehension to find out what he was going to say.

Then Mr Carmichael turned towards the nurse and whispered, "There is no staging on these notes." They both glanced at each other very quickly.

The nurse whispered back to him, "It's T4." Mr Carmichael immediately slumped in his chair and sighed.

I knew immediately what T4 meant. Colon cancer, like all cancers, is classified by four stages, ranging from 0-4, with the fourth stage being the most serious. T4 meant, effectively, the cancer will inevitably spread to other parts of her body.

Mum was completely oblivious as to the seriousness of her illness.

"We are going to keep you in for a few days," Mr Carmichael said gently to Mum.

"Can I go home first?" Mum asked in a quiet but hesitant voice. "I don't have any overnight clothes with me."

"You won't need them," he replied in his smooth, reassuring voice.

He then leaned forward and looked into Mum's eyes. "Mrs Carrington, I believe you have cancer of the colon. You have an extensive tumour. We need to carry out further examinations, but the initial test results indicate that the tumour is now malignant."

In terms of the precise clinical terminology, Mum had caecal adenocarcinoma with necrotic local nodes. The tumour was on her right side. Mr Carmichael advised the nurse that Mum required major surgery urgently.

"We will need to run further investigations—a CT scan on the abdominal and pelvis to see if it has spread into the blood stream. We will also look at your lymph nodes," Mr Carmichael commented sympathetically.

Staring at Mum straight into her eyes, Mr Carmichael whispered "you need to be admitted immediately. You are malnourished and anaemic. You need an urgent blood transfusion."

The consultation lasted less than ten minutes.

We were then led out of the room. We sat in a corridor with a long row of seats. It was crowded, but all I remember is that we felt so alone. Mum looked so shocked. She began to cry. I couldn't recall seeing Mum cry before in my life.

I tried to reassure and console her and told her everything was going to be all right. "We will get through this," I kept saying to her, but inside, I was in pieces. As we were waiting, I realised Mum had incurable cancer. It felt like a great burden had been laid on my heart, and I felt so alone and completely helpless with this devastating news.

My heart was simultaneously filled up with so much love and overwhelming sorrow for her.

Another two hours passed. We were still sitting in the corridor, waiting to be told what ward Mum needed to be admitted to. Then a senior ward manager came round and informed us that they didn't have any beds available in the hospital. We were advised the nearest neighbouring hospital was the King Edward Hospital, which was about ten miles away. The nurse refused to provide an ambulance to take us there. I was all ready to complain. Mum pleaded with me in her breathless voice. "Mark, I don't want any fuss, please do not complain." So we caught a taxi outside the hospital reception. We arrived at the King Edward Hospital, Accident and Emergency Department around 4:30 pm. It was a stifling hot day. To my total astonishment, the Accident and Emergency Department was overflowing with people, noisy and chaotic. It was full of people who were inebriated. I could see immediately that it was a hostile environment.

A seemingly innocuous incident between a man and a woman queuing up at the reception desk suddenly turned into a violent altercation between them. The police were called and the matter was eventually cleared up.

It was so crowded that all the seats were taken in the waiting area. Mum could hardly stand up. She was clinging on to me tightly. I even had to ask a young man to give up his seat for Mum. He did so begrudgingly. I simply could not understand how St John's Hospital sent us down to the Accident and Emergency Department of a neighbouring hospital, in the full knowledge that Mum had been diagnosed with advanced cancer. She was in total shock. She could hardly walk and needed medical attention and a hospital bed urgently.

We finally saw the triage doctor at 6:30 pm. A full two hours since we arrived. When we entered the cubicle, the triage doctor started to speak sharply and abruptly to Mum. I immediately interrupted in the attempt to correct the doctor's behaviour. "Please don't talk to my Mum like that. You can see she is extremely frail." I said annoyingly.

22

"Don't you have any notes?" I enquired. "No," the doctor replied. Before we left St John's hospital, I was assured Mum's notes would be forwarded on. Clearly this had not happened.

I explained that, earlier in the day, we had attended St John's Hospital where Mum had been diagnosed with Stage 4 colon cancer and she urgently needed a blood transfusion. "She shouldn't be in the Accident and Emergency Department," I demanded. This cut no ice with the triage doctor. "You just have to wait your turn," she retorted. "You can see there are hundreds of people that need to be seen before you. Just take a look, they are waiting in the corridors to be seen."

Surely, I argued, a cancer patient should be seen immediately. "The only way you can be allocated a bed in this hospital is by two routes. By referral only from your consultant. Alternatively, you come to us through Accident and Emergency," she commented tersely. "I'm afraid you just have to wait."

We walked back out to the waiting area. All the seats were made of metal and were extremely uncomfortable. I then asked the receptionist if she had a pillow for Mum to sit on. "No," she replied unapologetically. "What about a wheelchair?" I asked. "We don't have any in the Accident and Emergency Department," the receptionist grumbled. The receptionist was completely uncooperative.

As I walked back to Mum, I put my coat on her seat to make it more comfortable for her.

A further three hours passed before she saw a consultant doctor. As Mum was shunted into a small cubicle, we walked passed an elderly man on a hospital trolley, seemingly waiting to be treated. He looked in agony.

Then we passed a woman who was visibly intoxicated. She was shouting and ripping off her monitoring equipment.

Over the next few hours, Mum saw a series of junior consultants. They were all very pleasant and kind to her. She had no idea what was going on. I had to explain the events of the day to each doctor who came round to examine her.

I was then asked to ring St John's Hospital and request for them to forward Mum's notes. I finally managed to contact Mr Carmichael. He apologised for the confusion.

The lack of communication and coordination was evident.

Thankfully, by 10:30 pm, after hours of waiting, Mum was settled in a medical ward in the King Edward Hospital. I was so relieved. She desperately needed a blood transfusion.

Once Mum was settled in the ward, one of the nurses decided to take some blood from her.

First she tried Mum's right arm. Mum pointed out that she wouldn't find any blood there, but the nurse wouldn't listen to her. Mum was right. After ten minutes, the nurse stopped, leaving Mum's arm covered with bruises. Mum shouted, "You had punched me. You are not going to do that to me again." The nurse left angrily. Through her body language, I could see she had no compassion for the patients on the ward. I subsequently complained to the Matron, who was more sympathetic. Thankfully, she took over trying to take blood from Mum. She too could not find a vein. Then, suddenly, in a eureka-like moment, Matron yelled, "I've found one. That is a nice vein." Mum rolled her eyes as if to say, *did you have to find it?*

3

Gathering my thoughts and feelings

I left Mum that evening and headed back home. I arrived home around 11pm.

As I walked in the house, all her possessions were scattered around the living room, exactly how we had left them 12 hours before. Her glasses were lying on the sofa. Her cup was on the table. Her jumper, all folded up neatly, was lying on the back of her chair and her front door keys were lying on the windowsill. I suddenly felt totally numb. Our home for 21 years had always been warm, friendly, and full of love. It now seemed stone cold without her.

It is hard to express how I felt that day. It was an unbelievable shock. The news was devastating. I felt like someone had just grabbed my world and turned it upside down. It was as if the axis had come off the wheels of my life. I knew that from now on, my life would be different.

Words in themselves will never be enough to articulate the deep emotions I went through that day. I felt so powerless.

I remember that night vividly. It was 2 am as I was lying in bed. I simply couldn't move. I started having a panic attack. First, my heart started beating irregularly. This was shortly followed by sweating and shaking. My whole body began to tremble. I felt nauseous and started to heave. My chest was tightening up. A minute seemed like an hour. I was in total shock and agony. It felt like someone had just punched me in the stomach not just once, but over a hundred times.

I managed to crawl to the bathroom, where I vomited copiously for about an hour. I then sat on the bathroom floor, unable to move. I was just sobbing uncontrollably. I finally managed to stumble back to bed at about 4 am.

My body was reacting to the enormity of the news. There was a profound realisation that Mum, unless a miracle were to happen, was going to die.

I simply don't know how I managed to get through that night. But somehow I did. As the morning slowly broke, I saw the bright glowing sunrise. I decided to take a shower and cooked myself breakfast.

There was no question about looking after Mum. To me, Mum came first and last. That evening, I made a silent promise to myself that I would look after her. I made a conscious decision to be the rock by her side. But I was consumed with fear, not only for Mum, but fear about my own ability. I kept asking myself, *am I capable of looking after Mum?* I had no idea what laid in front of me. I was in a complete void. Then something got hold of me. I knew I had to be a different person. That night, I sat down and wrote out a charter. I was determined to follow it every day.

I pinned it up on my bedroom wall. It read:

- I recognise and accept that it is Mum's illness. It is her body. And ultimately, it is her journey.
- I will not grieve while Mum is still alive.
- I will cherish and remember all the beautiful and spontaneous moments we have together during her illness.
- I will be Mum's advocate as she proceeds through the healthcare system. I will fight for her with every last breath I have. I am determined that she will not live in distress.
- I will preserve Mum's dignity to the end.
- I will focus on Mum's physical and mental well-being and not entirely on what the medical profession tells us.
- I will support Mum's right to mental and physical independence, by encouraging her to do as much as she can

for herself while giving her support when she needs it. I will treat Mum normally and not be too overprotective so that she loses her independence.

- I will ensure that at all times Mum will not feel like she is a burden, which from my perspective she never has been.
- I will focus on one day at a time and only focus on what needs to be achieved on that day. I remember a saying from President Franklin D. Roosevelt, who insightfully said "Yesterday is history. Tomorrow is a mystery. But today is a gift, that is why it is called the present." In other words, live in the moment.

Above all else, as Mum was always a loving and caring woman, I was determined to ensure that the cancer was not going to rob her of her identity as a person and steal her independence.

I hoped the charter was going to help me. But little did I know then how powerful and life-affirming it was going to be.

After my body had recovered from the shock of the news, I had some really big decisions to make. I knew the hardest thing to witness in my life was to watch Mum's inevitable physical deterioration. As well as being a son, I was now Mum's carer and advocate. I knew she would be totally reliant on me. Never in my entire life had Mum not been there for me. She told me once that life does not come without sacrifice. It was now my turn to give something back to her. I never thought of or looked upon caring for Mum as a burden. It didn't even cross my mind. I viewed it as a beautiful and precious gift and I was so grateful that I was in a position to care for her.

My faith, which always spoke deeply inside me and brought healing to my heart, was going to be tested. I knew this was the time when I had to put into practice all the wisdom I had accumulated throughout my life.

Nevertheless, seeds of self-doubt kept creeping into my mind. Night after night, I started to agonise and torture myself as to whether I was capable for caring for Mum. No one gives you a road map about caring for someone you love who is dying. Night after night I would ruminate, repeatedly talking to myself. *I don't know where to start. I don't know if I am good enough. Will I let Mum down? Will I fail?* A dear friend said to me, "Mark, you can only do what you can do."

One night, I was reminiscing and drawing on all the events in my life, when I remembered one day at school back in the 1960s. My school arranged a day out to visit an old people's home. I talked to many old people about their lives, but one conversation stuck in my memory. It was with an elderly man called Jim. He told me about the atrocities that happened in Bergen-Belsen, the Nazi concentration camp in the Second World War. The camp was liberated in April 1945 by the British 11th Armoured Division.

He told me that no one deserved to witness what he had seen. There were approximately 50,000 prisoners inside, most of them half-starved and seriously ill, in addition to another 13,000 prisoners who died in the weeks after liberation. Corpses were lying around the camp unburied.

Then he told me a story of a simple act of kindness and goodness. He said that out of nowhere, a large amount of lipstick had arrived at the camp. It was an action of pure genius by an American General. Nothing did more for the internees than the lipstick. He described how he saw women with nothing but a blanket over their shoulders, now had scarlet lips. "I saw a woman dead on the table," he remembered, "and clutched in her hands was a tube of lipstick."

He then pointed out, looking straight into my eyes: "Don't you see, Mark, at last they were someone, not merely a number tattooed on their backs."

Our conversation had a profound effect on me. This seemingly small act of human kindness of giving lipstick to the female internees gave them back their femininity, dignity, and their sense of humanity.

He told me that a drop of human kindness costs nothing. He then told me something I will never forget. A person's dignity comes from their self-worth.

Drawing on this story and applying it to my situation, I promised myself that above all, I was going to do whatever I could to ensure Mum was cared for in a manner that preserved her dignity. While she was my mother, she was also a human being. I promised myself that through acts of kindness and love, cancer would not rob her of her identity and her femininity.

The next morning, I was on my way to the King Edward Hospital to see Mum, when I saw a homeless man sitting just outside the entrance of the hospital. He was finishing off what looked like a bottle of vodka. I looked into his eyes. They seemed strangely familiar and warm. For some reason, I stopped. He asked, "Do you wish to buy the Big Issue, sir?"

"Okay," I replied, as I was sorting out my loose change.

We started chatting. He told me that he had lost his wife to cancer in 2007. He subsequently fell apart, and then, due to the financial crash in 2008, he lost his house and had been homeless ever since. He explained he couldn't handle the real world so he chose to be homeless.

In all honesty, I was half listening to him. Because I was in so much distress, I wasn't taking too much notice of what he was saying.

He could see, however, the emotional pain on my face. "You are in pain. I can tell," he thoughtfully commented. I subsequently told him what happened to Mum. We prayed together. Then he gave some profound advice that I would never forget:

"Mark, listen to me. You must be strong. You must be strong with faith. You must be strong with the strength of hope. You must be strong with love that is stronger than death."

As I left him to go into the hospital, he quoted from the poet Mary Oliver. "To truly live in this world, you need to do three things: to love what is mortal, to hold it against your bones, knowing your whole life depends on it. And when the time comes, let it go. You will know when it is time to let go—it will be in your own time and at your own pace. Follow your heart and you will never go wrong. Your heart will tell you what to do."

I gave him some money and proceeded to go through the revolving doors into the hospital's atrium. I stopped just as I was inside and turned around and waved goodbye. He smiled and waved back.

The hospital receptionist could see I was startled. She immediately called over the security guard. And he moved the homeless person on. I protested to the security guard, arguing he was not harming anyone. But it was all to no avail. The heavy-handedness was all too apparent. The ruthlessness of how the guard dealt with this vulnerable man was totally shocking.

Then the homeless man shouted out to me. "Don't worry about me, Mark, I am used to it. You just look after your mum, she is the most important person in your life right now."

The lifts were out-of-order at the end of the corridor, so instead, I rushed up six flights of stairs to see Mum. I finally found her on the ward. "How are you? Did you sleep well?" I asked.

"No, I did not," she replied, seemingly annoyed. "The nurses kept on waking me up through the night. Checking this, checking that. I just want to go home."

I told her she needed to stay in the hospital for a few more days to get better. As I left Mum in the hospital that evening, on my way out, in the reception area, I dropped to my hands and knees and started vomiting. Again, it was my body reacting to the devastating news. Fortunately, I managed to rush over to a waste paper bin. No one helped or assisted me.

Eventually, after five days in the King Edward Hospital, Mum was discharged. She looked slightly better after the blood transfusion, but she still looked frail and malnourished.

The oncologist doctor set the operation to remove the tumour for three weeks' time.

Mum arrived home by taxi. Due to her illness, we had to make some further changes to our living arrangements. Mum continued to sleep downstairs on the sofa, with a pillow and a blanket to keep her warm.

One night, however, while I was sleeping, I heard a loud bang. I rushed downstairs and saw Mum on the floor. She had rolled off the sofa. I grabbed her and managed to lift and carry her back to the sofa. Fortunately, she hadn't hurt herself. I wrapped the blanket around her. She slept well that night.

At this stage, Mum was very weak. I weighed her and she was under six stone.

Mum was rapidly deteriorating. I had never seen her so weak and frail. To me, she looked like she was shortly going to pass away.

Being fiercely independent, Mum was adamant not to have carers in the house. She did not want strangers to look after her. She just wanted me.

Given her frailty, she was still lucid and made a compelling case that we only needed to wait three weeks until the operation and therefore, to bring carers in the house, would be pointless. I reluctantly agreed.

With our worlds turned up-side-down, our lives were in complete turmoil. We had no structure to our day. I quickly decided to put a daily routine together which focused on making sure Mum was both eating and constantly hydrated throughout the day. I felt helpless but that was all I could do.

In the mornings, I would cook porridge for breakfast. In terms of personal hygiene, I would bring Mum a bowl of warm water for bathing. She managed to wash and dress without my assistance.

On occasions, I would wash her back. I could see her bones sheering through her skin. As I washed her, tears would be running down my face, but I was careful for her not to see I was crying. To witness, in front of my eyes, the sheer and utter vulnerability of another human being was both shocking and deeply profound. It was an immense privilege and responsibility caring for someone so vulnerable.

I would also wash her feet, cut her toenails and massage her legs with moisturising cream. She allowed me on one occasion to cut her hair.

Mum was too weak to even flush the toilet. So we agreed that I would flush it for her. Without her knowing, it gave me the opportunity to check her urine and poo for any signs of blood. I didn't see any. I also checked her urine colour to see if she was hydrated throughout the day.

She kept on saying to me, "I'm so sorry you have to do this. I do appreciate your help. Thank you."

I would reply to her reassuringly, "You don't ever need to thank me. I'm your son."

Regarding daily chores, I would go out and do the shopping every day. I would cry spontaneously as I was walking down the street. The tears would be flowing down my face to such an extent that the tears stung my eyes.

As I was doing the ironing, washing up, or even vacuuming the house, I would pray for Mum. Having my own silent time with God, gave me personal solace and strength during this period of my life.

We somehow managed to get through each day.

4

First operation

Four weeks had passed in an instant. It was now Monday, 14th July 2014, the day of Mum's operation.

It was pitch dark, cold, and drizzling with rain as we arrived at the King Edward Hospital at 7 am. There was no one around. Then, at around 7:30 am, the receptionist rushed through the door. She took her coat off and began to log on to her computer. It took about 20 minutes before she finally found Mum's name on the system and allocated her a time for the operation. We were then told to wait in a small room. As we waited, Mum became increasingly anxious and distraught. As much as I could, I tried to reassure her that everything was going to be alright.

At around 8 am, we saw the senior surgeon who was going to perform Mum's operation. He was very cordial and professional. He had a soft and warm voice that managed to put Mum at ease. He could see instantly that Mum was extremely nervous. He told Mum that she was in very capable hands. "We have an excellent team of surgeons that are going to look after you," he pledged to her in a comforting voice.

He was honest and sensitive as he explained to Mum the purpose of her operation and the morbidity risk of the surgery, which in Mum's case was extremely high due to her severe weight loss and lack of muscle tone. He stressed that all he could do was his best. I thanked him and accepted that was all I could hope for.

He was overjoyed as he managed to arrange Mum's operation to be his first of the day.

Mum was then asked to sign a consent form. She did so without hesitation. She fully understood the risks involved. He asked Mum whether she wanted her organs to be donated. She didn't mind, and, subsequently, agreed. The surgeon commented that all her organs were healthy, ironically; it was just the tumour that was the problem. As we left the room, Mum thanked him.

We were then told to wait in a smaller waiting room. Suddenly, the room filled with other women waiting for their operations on the same day. Some were there for ankle and knee operations. They were all talking, laughing, and giggling with each other. Mum, by now a frail-looking woman, was just sitting there, gazing into space. She looked so frightened and scared. I just could not believe that Mum was having a major operation, which she might not survive, while surrounded by lively and much younger women who were preparing for their minor operations. It simply didn't seem right.

Then the nurse walked in the room. She looked at me. "You are not allowed to be here," she advised sternly. "This is a women's only room."

Mum clutched my hand. "I am looking after my Mum," I replied. The nurse reassured me that she would be fine without me. Mum obviously did not want me to leave, but I simply had no choice.

As I walked out the door, I glanced back. I saw Mum sitting on a hard metal seat looking so frightened and vulnerable. I waved to her. My heart sank as I closed the door behind me.

As I left, I asked the doctor when I should return. "I should say around 3:30 pm," he replied.

In my heart of hearts, I felt that I needed to be close to Mum during her operation. I simply couldn't leave the hospital building. Fortunately, the hospital had a canteen on the ground floor. So I decided to have breakfast there.

Time passed so quickly. My mobile phone rang about 10:30 am when I was in the process of digesting my breakfast.

I quickly answered the call.

A nurse answered the phone.

"Is that Mark Carrington?"

"Yes," I replied.

"The son of Marian Carrington?"the voice added.

Before I could answer, my heart had sunk.

"Yes," I responded.

"I am one of the nurses looking after your mother. I would just like to let you know that your mother is fine. It is just that we are unable to operate as we do not have a bed for her," she whispered.

I rushed to see Mum immediately. She was sitting on a bed in a small cubicle, looking so dejected. She asked me not to make a fuss. But I couldn't let this go. After numerous conversations with the nurses, I simply couldn't get an answer. So I demanded to see the senior consultant.

"Are you seriously telling me you cannot allocate a bed for my Mum?" I argued. "The operation was planned four weeks ago. Are you telling me that you are unable to find a bed for a patient who has advanced cancer and requires an urgent operation?"

He apologised. He explained it was out of his hands as it was the bed manager's responsibility to allocate beds each day.

After an hour of arguing, a bed was finally assigned for Mum. It was now 12:30 pm. I was asked to leave quickly. Both Mum and I had no chance to say goodbye, but we managed to wave to each other quickly before the doctor closed the door abruptly.

I decided to stay in the hospital's canteen all day. In total, I probably drank about fifteen cups of tea. I had my mobile phone on throughout the day, but it didn't even ring once.

Five o'clock passed. Six o'clock passed. By seven o'clock, I still hadn't received a phone call. After waiting eight or nine hours, I still didn't know if the operation had been a success or not. Finally, I decided to run up the stairs to the sixth floor where Mum's operation was taking place.

When I reached the floor, the corridor was empty, with no one in sight. I started to pace up and down the passageway, hoping against hope I would see someone who could tell me news about my Mum. Then by chance, as if fate would have it, a door opened. It so happened to be the surgeon we saw earlier in the day.

"Don't you know, Mark?" he enquired.

"Know what?" I replied hesitantly. He sat me down. For the second time in the day. My heart sank.

"Your mum is fine," he announced in his softly spoken voice.

Before he could finish his sentence, I screamed, "Thank you, God."

"But the procedure did not go to plan," he continued. "We had to stop the operation and resuscitate your mum. Mark, your mum had a severe allergic reaction. Although we are not certain, we believe it might have been the intravenous line inserted in her, which was coated with chlorhexidine. We simply don't know yet. He concluded.

"Her heart rate increased," he added. "Her heart was palpitating. Her blood pressure had decreased. The whole of her left arm became all purple. After five hours, we decided the best course of action was not to operate. Do you know that we even had to cancel the whole day's operations?"

I felt a sense of relief she was alright, but then, that relief turned into the realisation that we were no further forward, and Mum was still facing a traumatic time ahead. She still had the tumour inside her, which needed to be removed. She was also still frail and malnourished.

I was in no fit state to see Mum that evening. I was still in shock and extremely emotional receiving the news as to what had happened to her. Also I had to gather my thoughts on what we both had to face. So I headed home.

The next morning, I arrived at the hospital about 9 am. When I reached the ward, Mum was sitting up having breakfast. She was complaining that her toast was cold. I smiled. I was pleased she was moaning. I told her that she would still moan even if she were living in Buckingham Palace. That made her smile.

"They told me what happened when I came around from the anaesthetic," she said surprisingly. "I thought it was a bit strange as I wasn't in any pain."

I laughed.

Mum was given a blood transfusion and was allowed to stay in the hospital over the course of the weekend.

Before she was discharged, the surgeon arranged Mum's surgery. "It will be another six weeks, I'm afraid," he said apologetically.

"Is that the earliest you can operate on Mum?" I asked.

"Yes. In any event, I am going away for a three-week holiday in the Seychelles," he professed.

He then reassured me, however, that the tumour would not grow substantially in that period and that Mum would not deteriorate.

5

Homecoming

Still frail and weak, Mum was discharged on Monday. We arrived home by taxi around 4 pm.

The next six weeks were going to be difficult. Despite her frailties, Mum was still insistent she didn't require any care support. She was determined not to have strangers in her home. Even at this stage of her illness, she was fiercely guarding her independence.

I was nearly at breaking point. So I had to be completely honest and told her that I did not think I could cope caring for on my own. After a long conversation, Mum agreed, albeit reluctantly, for a carer to visit twice a day – to wash her and prepare lunch. The next day, I contacted our local council to arrange for the appropriate care provision to be put in place.

The following Monday, a carer started. Her name was Julie. She was amiable, caring, and friendly. Each day she would arrive at the house promptly at 9 am to wash Mum and then return around 1 pm to help with Mum's lunch.

Over the course of Julie's first week, she encouraged me to go out, so I could spend quality time with my friends in the sound knowledge that she would be looking after Mum. She would spend hours with Mum.

Then one day as I returned home, I walked into the living room and there in front of me was Julie on her knees praying in front of Mum. Mum looked up at me and explained that Julie had been preaching and trying to convert her to a different religion. I immediately looked across the room and saw our coffee table covered in religious literature.

I immediately thanked Julie for praying for Mum. I firmly explained, however, that her behaviour was unacceptable and fundamentally breached the code of conduct for adult social care. I graciously told her never to return. That afternoon, I reported the incident to the local authority.

Fortunately, Mum saw the funny side of it: "Mark, all your life you have been trying to convert me to vote Conservative (Mum was a lifelong Labour supporter), now you are attempting to change my religion too." We both laughed. The incident put a smile on Mum's face as I tucked her into bed that evening.

As a result of this episode, Mum did not want any further carers in the house before her operation. Given what happened, I could understand her reason. Therefore, the responsibility for caring for Mum would lay solely with me. I would wash and keep Mum clean. She would constantly look at her arms and cry that they were wrinkled, and in her words, looked like alligator skin.

My immediate concern was to guard Mum against any exposure to negativity. I understood that the most basic human needs of any of us are to be safe, to be secure and to be loved. In silent contemplation, I made a promise to myself to protect her and ensure no one was going to harm her.

At this point, as Mum was more frailer both physically and mentally, there was a real danger that she could easily get caught in an emotional downward spiral of always worrying. Observing her behaviour pattern, it was clear that even the slightest problem or incident would agitate her. For example, when we received letters through the post, she worried that they were bills to be paid and whether we had enough money to pay them.

In terms of our day-to-day practical living arrangements, it was imperative I reduced Mum's anxiety. This, in effect, meant ensuring all our bills were paid on time and we always had sufficient food in the house. I kept reassuring her that she did not need to worry about our finances. Day after day, I tried to put her mind at ease. I kept reassuring her that the only person she needed to focus on was herself.

We both agreed that she would not answer the phone when I was out of the house as at the time, we were receiving numerous nuisance calls. For example, we were receiving calls from companies selling insurance policies. Such calls only served to increase her anxiety and stress.

Given the circumstances, I knew rushing back to work would have been a mistake. It was imperative that I maximised the time I had with Mum at home. As I already used my annual leave entitlement, I agreed with my employer to take a further twelve weeks' unpaid leave. My employer was satisfied with that arrangement, as I knew they didn't want me to return to work.

Over the course of my career, I understood how power struggles manifest themselves within organisations. They are part of office politics. With Mum having cancer, it gave my employer the perfect opportunity to reorganise me out of my job. As I had only been working there for just under two years, I had no employment rights. At that particular point in my life, however, work was a secondary consideration. My entire focus was on caring for Mum.

After the first operation, the doctors at the King Edward Hospital wanted to know precisely what caused Mum's allergic reaction. In particular, the surgeons were desperate to avoid a repeat of the incident. So, during the next six weeks, Mum was subjected to numerous allergy tests. After an exhaustive round of assessments, the doctors, however, could still not pinpoint the precise reason. The best conclusion they came up with was that it was indeed the chlorhexidine that was given to her through the tube.

On Mum's final appointment, I started to chat to the senior allergy consultant. She told me that she was currently caring for her mum as well. She understood and could empathise with what I was going through. "Your mum is delightful," she told me in a tender tone. "She resonates remarkable warmth. Even in the face of adversity. Your mum has a strength of character and a wonderful spirit."

"I know," I replied with a warm glow in my eyes, "I am very lucky." We hugged. I then kissed her hand. I thanked her for all the help she was giving Mum and wished her well with looking after her own mother.

Two weeks before the operation, Mum was also asked to attend a memory clinic at the hospital. Initially, Mum was reluctant, which was typical of her, but after some cajoling, she finally agreed.

We arrived at the hospital at 2 pm. As we were waiting in reception, a junior consultant greeted Mum.

"I am Dr Phillips," she announced. "I am the junior doctor who will be assessing you today. Before you undertake the assessment, I would like you to draw a clock on a piece of paper." She immediately walked back to her office. We waited a further hour before a Mum's name was called out over the loud speaker. We were then led into a small room. As we walked in, Dr Phillips was sitting down writing some notes. She looked up and asked Mum what time she had drawn on the clock face.

"Seven o'clock," Mum replied. "Anyone can see that. I am not out of my mind just yet."

I explained to Dr Phillips that we were not advised that a memory assessment was going to be conducted. I told her that Mum was exhausted and I did not think she was ready or prepared for the assessment. Dr Phillips simply shrugged her shoulders and proceeded with further memory exercises.

"Where do you live?" she asked.

Mum told her the address.

"Where is that?" Dr Phillips enquired.

"Fulham," Mum asserted.

Dr Phillips probed further, "Where is Fulham?"

"What kind of a question is that?" Mum replied, looking perplexed.

Using a different tack, Dr Phillips enquired, "Where is this hospital?"

"Paddington," Mum replied confidently.

Frustratingly, Dr Phillips looked at me and fumed, "We are not getting very far with these questions."

"Do you know what day it is today?" quizzed Dr Phillips.

"Yes," Mum responded.

"Would you like to tell me then?" Dr Phillips retorted while sighing heavily.

"Why, don't you know?" Mum whispered innocently.

Mum was not being difficult. Her hearing was not good. She was doing her very best to answer the questions. But at this stage, Dr Phillips was getting increasingly annoyed. It was evident to me, as the tests carried on, that Dr Phillips failed to grasp how much information Mum could digest.

She raised her voice. "Okay, what month is it? Can you tell me the days of the week backwards?"

Mum smiled. She recounted the days with ease.

Dr Phillips then proceeded to go through a different checklist of questions. She explained that the questions were designed to determine whether Mum was depressed or not.

"What are your goals in life?"

Mum and I glanced at each other.

"What do you want to be doing in five years' time?"

Dr Phillips proceeded with a further ten questions.

I looked on in total astonishment as she read question after question from the checklist.

At the end of the consultation, Dr Phillips concluded that Mum was suffering from depression.

Mum was extremely sad and apprehensive but in my opinion, not depressed. We left the room stunned.

Two weeks later, Mum subsequently received a letter from the hospital. It stated:

"This lady has a depressive affect and scored 11/30 on the geriatric depression scale. This is suggestive of a depressive episode and may explain a score of 7/30 on the Montreal Cognitive

Assessment. It is likely there is an underlying cognitive disorder. There is a high risk of postoperative dysfunction, delirium, and cognitive decline. This lady will need a permanent care home. It is unlikely she will ever have a balance of mind to exercise any rational decisions regarding her care provision."

I simply could not believe what I was reading. How on earth could a junior doctor make such a clinical judgement, especially based on only one round of tests? The assessment was lamentable, poor, and weak. If Mum were by herself with no advocate by her side, based on this flimsy evaluation, she would have been shunted quickly away, out of sight, in a care home.

I was in the process of making a formal complaint, but Mum, once again, did not want any fuss. So I left the matter. I focused all my energies once again on caring for Mum.

Over the coming six weeks, I could see Mum was deteriorating further. She looked more anaemic, frailer, and more anorexic. She still looked extremely malnourished. By the beginning of August 2014, she weighed only five and a half stone. I felt totally helpless and powerless.

Over and over again, I asked myself, as a son, how I could have allowed her to get like this. Night after night, I went to sleep guilt-ridden for letting this happen to her under my care. While I realised it was, in fact, the tumour inside her that was causing her malnourishment, I still felt I was to blame. At the time, I felt I let Mum down. And to some extent, I still do even today.

Mum and I continued with our daily routine. I read my charter on a daily basis—it always gave me focus and solace. During the six weeks leading up to the operation, Mum became increasingly anxious, scared, and agitated. Every time I went to the bathroom, she would shout out to me to hurry back. Each time I came back home from shopping, she fretted that I had taken too long.

On one occasion, I was upstairs in my bedroom. Mum went to use the toilet downstairs. Then, a minute after, I heard her screaming. I ran down the stairs. She physically couldn't get up from the raised toilet seat. I rushed upstairs to the main bathroom and grabbed a large bath towel.

Then I managed to wrap the towel around her to ensure her dignity was preserved. I started to lift her up slowly and gently with her arms wrapped around my upper body. I carried her into the living room whereby I eased her down into her chair. She was utterly distraught. It took me all evening to calm her down.

Fortunately, I was in the house at the time to help her. That night, I kept on thinking about the incident. What if the incident occurred when I was out shopping? I agonised every time I left the house. Every day, a whole range of emotions and fears would pass through my head.

The weeks passed in a flash.

6

Main operation

Mum attended a routine consultation with a junior anaesthetist, precisely a week before her surgery to remove her tumour.

At this point, Mum's mobility was extremely poor. Her weight loss was very visible, dramatic, and extremely disturbing. Losing more weight, she was now close to weighing five stone. It was clear to me she was now suffering from the acute form of cachexia (which is prevalent in people with advanced colon cancer). Cachexia is a body syndrome that causes anorexia, and it cannot be reversed nutritionally.

In Mum's case, she had lost both her lean and skeleton muscle mass as a direct result of the solid, malignant tumour inside her.

During the consultation, the junior anaesthetist was blunt and direct. "We have no choice but to operate, Mrs Carrington," he explained. "Please be under no illusion, this is a major operation you are facing. If we do not remove the tumour, you will die very quickly, probably in a few weeks. If we, however, operate, because of your lack of muscle tissue and tone, you will be at high risk, and it is highly likely that you will not come through the surgery."

Spontaneously, without any warning, the junior anaesthetist leaned across and touched Mum's hand and whispered, "Your body will need to fight like never before for you to survive the surgery."

Mum looked numbed. She was put in an impossible

situation. The junior anaesthetist agreed that Mum needed a further blood transfusion, but insisted that she could only stay in the hospital for one night. Mum protested, as she wanted to go home. But it was for the best. I left Mum to settle on the ward before I headed home.

That night, I simply couldn't sleep. I kept ruminating and thinking what a dreadful situation for anyone to be in, let alone my mother. She was unlikely to survive the operation in the physical state she was in. The balance of risk was around 95 percent against her surviving, primarily due to her extreme weight loss and lack of muscle. I was determined to tilt that balance so she had, at least, a fighting chance of survival.

Once again, I looked at my charter. I repeated to myself, "I will fight for Mum with every breath I have. She has no one else on her side."

The next day, at 9 am, I decided to see the senior consultant, Mr Michael Bucannon, at the King Edward Hospital. While I didn't have an appointment to see him, I found out the location of his office. I spoke to his secretary, who thankfully, allowed me to see him for five minutes during the day. My prayer was answered. I knew that was all I needed.

When I met him, I made a cogent, coherent, and compelling case that Mum not only needed to be kept in hospital, but to be also intravenously fed with nutrition to build her up ready for the surgery.

Mr Bucannon listened intently. Thankfully, my argument prevailed and he agreed with me. I subsequently had to break the news to Mum that she was to stay in the hospital for the lead up to her operation. She so desperately wanted to come home. At the time, I didn't tell her that it was my idea.

On that same day, the nurses hooked Mum up to a feeding drip. She was fed intravenously through the nose for twenty-four hours a day, right up to the day of her operation. The plan worked. She put on nine pounds in five days. I was so relieved. She was now at least given a fighting chance, no matter how slim. I accepted that if she died on the operating table, I knew in my heart I tried my best for her.

Mum was annoyed and would repeatedly say to me, "I don't want to be here, I don't want the drip through my nose. I don't want any fuss made over me." I told her that we were never going to stop 'fussing' over her whether she liked it or not.

Over the course of the week, Mum started to have a glow in her face. On the day of the surgery, I arrived on the ward to see her at 7 am. She was calm and relaxed but tearful. I was only allowed to spend about ten minutes with her. As she was being wheeled to the theatre, I managed to wave her goodbye. She smiled and waved back. As I left the ward, I wondered to myself if that was going to be the last time I would see Mum alive. I still needed to feel I was close to her during her operation. So, once again, I headed to the hospital's canteen.

As I queued up to purchase a cappuccino by the cashier's counter, I suddenly turned around. I simply could not believe my eyes. There standing next to me, was Mr Bucannon. He seemed relaxed.

"Don't worry, your mum will be fine," he testified proudly. "She is in safe hands. I am going to be in charge of your mum's operation. We are going to have two anaesthetists present in the theatre, just in case something goes wrong. Do you know she has put on nine pounds since being intravenously fed?" he announced triumphantly.

I stayed in the hospital canteen all day. I must have drunk another fifteen cups of tea. I was a complete bag of nerves. I prayed all day. Prayer was all I had. The senior nurse promised me that she would ring me on my mobile phone at the end of the day. It was like Groundhog Day. No one rang.

By 8 pm, I could wait no longer. I was at my wit's end. I subsequently phoned the ward nurse. She calmly explained that the operation lasted nine hours and was mostly a success. The tumour was longer than the doctors expected. It was not only 12 centimetres long—more than twice the size when it was measured in June when they took the MRI scan—but it also weighed one and half pounds. I could not believe how a tumour could be so long and weigh so much. She told me that Mum had been transferred to the high-dependency unit.

The next day, I visited Mum around 3:30 pm. But, curiously, she wasn't there. I asked the nurse on the ward as to her whereabouts. She informed me that she had been taken down for an X-ray. I was then asked to wait in a small waiting room. Some three hours passed. I kept on thinking that it seemed a long time to take an X-ray.

Suddenly, Mr Bucannon walked through the door. I immediately knew something was wrong.

"Mark… sit down,"Mr Bucannon asserted. My heart sank again.

"Your mum has suffered a major setback," he calmly informed me. "We discovered that the stent we left in her body from yesterday's operation had leaked. We needed to carry out further surgery urgently."

He explained that he would be investigating the matter as it was extremely unusual and was probably caused by a manufacturer's malfunction. My reaction was of complete shock.

But he reassured me that Mum was in a stable condition. That was the only thing that mattered to me. I had to wait a further 24 hours to see if she would come through the second operation. Thankfully, she did. I decided not to see Mum that evening as I was conscious that she needed to rest. So I headed home.

The next morning, I headed back up to the hospital.

To the surprise of the doctors, Mum was sitting up. I just arrived as the nurses were giving her paracetamol.

Around dinner time, one of the nurses gave Mum a small bowl of soup. "It tastes dreadful," Mum commented. "It is so salty."

"You need to eat it," the nurse replied sternly.

"If it is so good, why don't you have it yourself?" Mum retorted.

The nurse looked stunned that a patient would talk back to her. To me, it was another demonstration that Mum still had fight and spirit in her. I smiled.

Then Mum wanted to scratch her leg. She was wearing very tight bed socks to stop any blood clotting, but she had this insatiable itch, so I pulled off her socks.

Mum was also eager to show me her scars. In fact, she was quite proud of them. "Look," she said boastfully. "They stapled in the stitches."

She insisted on showing them to me. As I was squeamish, I just had one quick glance.

"Before the operation, the doctor drew on me where the insertions were going to be made. I had all drawings on me," she said majestically.

She was moved out of the high-dependency unit after only two days. I was so relieved that she came through the operation. The doctors came around and told Mum the surgery was a success. The main tumour had been removed.

A few days later, however, the doctors thought Mum had pleural effusion—fluid on the lungs that would need to be drained by another operation. It appeared some fluid had collected between the sheets of tissue that cover the outside of her right lung and the lining of her chest cavity.

The doctors were deliberating on whether or not to operate. Thankfully, the decision was to monitor the situation rather than to operate. Personally, I didn't think Mum could have survived three major operations one after another within a few days.

Mum stayed in the hospital for five and a half weeks. During this time, I went to visit her every single day, both in the morning and in the afternoon. I worried about how she had slept or even if something dreadful had happened during the previous night. So I would always go up in the mornings to see her for about ten minutes. The Matron on the ward didn't seem to mind as long as I didn't stay too long.

I would then return in the afternoon and stay for a few hours. Mum worried that it was boring for me. I didn't mind. As long as Mum was okay, that was good enough for me. In fact, most of the time, I would just sit in a chair next to her.

We didn't need to speak. It was just nice to be by her side. She could feel my presence.

One afternoon, I looked across from Mum's bed. Opposite was an elderly woman who was crying out. She looked so vulnerable and debilitated.

I could see she had slumped in her bed. It appeared that she had slipped so far down that it was only a matter of time before she was going to fall onto the floor. I called for the nurses but there were none around. So I decided to walk over and lift her into the bed. She was extremely thankful for making her comfortable. She had a tearful expression on her face.

I noticed previously that, day after day, no one came to see her. She had no visitors. On this particular day, she had been left untended by the nurses for hours. I could not believe the level of her neglect. Later that day, I finally found the Matron and told her of my concerns.

Five days later, we discovered that the woman had suffered a stroke. The nurses had moved her to another ward. We never saw her again.

After my visits to Mum every morning and afternoon, it was clear that this particular ward was operating at or beyond its capacity. In my opinion, safety was being compromised because of this. It was plain to see that they were simply stretched and understaffed.

I was in the hospital all the time, arguing Mum's case, but I knew that many elderly people do not have family members by their side, just like the elderly woman opposite Mum's bed. She now had a real uphill struggle in life. Mum's words resonated with me: "By the grace of God go I." I'm always grateful for what I have in life because I know it can be taken away in an instant.

It was interesting to contrast the behaviour of the nurses in the different hospital wards Mum stayed in, even in the same hospital. In this particular ward, the nurses were stern and uncaring and Mum felt invisible. But on other wards, Mum could not have received better treatment—they treated her as if she was the only patient there.

Every week that Mum was laying in her bed, I could see her mentally deteriorating.

The warning signs of Mum developing delirium were all too apparent. For anyone who does not know what delirium is, it is an unforeseen and immediate disruption of a person's consciousness and cognition highlighted by vivid hallucinations, delusions, and an inability to focus.

Over the coming weeks, Mum became increasingly lethargic and inattentive. She was also losing weight again. Day after day, she would be resting in bed staring at a white wall. Her mind was completely inactive and her cognitive skills were decreasing. Worryingly, she started to hallucinate and on occasions was delusional. "I can see a black bird," she insisted as she pointed to the other bed across the ward. At this stage, I simply pacified her.

Then things turned for the worst. One Thursday, I arrived at the ward around 3:30pm.

Mum was sitting on her bed. She sat me down next to her. She looked at me straight in the eyes.

"Mark, listen to me, this is very serious," she said hesitantly. "I have swallowed two bugs. They are inside me crawling around. The doctors told me I don't have much time to live."

She was totally convinced. Her experience was totally real to her. As she spoke, her whole body was shaking. She was breathless. And her eyes were red. I could see she had been crying. I had never seen her so scared.

"The woman in the other bed has eaten one too," Mum added.

I knew straight away not to contradict her. I simply went with the flow of what she was saying. Listening intently, I rubbed her arm, trying to reassure her and calming her fears.

"I'm sure it will be fine," I replied tenderly with a tear running down my right eye.

I reported the incidents to the ward doctor.

"We can prescribe her antipsychotic medication to calm her down," he advised.

That was the last thing I wanted him to do, as I knew the

drugs might have made her worse and had serious side effects.

She was increasingly becoming more fearful. And with each day passing, losing her confidence. Somehow, I knew I had to get her out of the hospital and back home into her own environment. I could then look after her and start to stimulate her mentally.

But for now, the most important news was that the cancerous tissue was apparently gone.

Two weeks after the operation, however, the mood of the doctors changed. One morning, a senior surgeon examined Mum.

"Mrs Carrington, while we removed the tumour and that part of the operation was successful, there were some cells we couldn't remove. Do you understand what I am saying to you?"

"Yes," replied Mum apologetically. "Thank you for all your help."

She clutched his hand and wouldn't let it go.

It was Wednesday, 10th September 2014. I arrived at the hospital to see Mum at the usual time of 9 am. The junior doctor and the occupational therapist came around to see Mum. They drew the flimsy blue curtains around us.

"Marian, you haven't seen me before. I'm Dr Harding, a junior consultant. I have just recently joined the hospital."

Then Dr Harding held Mum's hands.

"Your hands are cold," Mum immediately commented.

"Marian, we feel you can go home now. How do you feel about that?" Dr Harding asked.

"Great," Mum said enthusiastically as her tiny eyes lit up.

I knew she desperately wanted to come home.

"Well, we'll sort out the discharge papers, and you can go home on Friday."

I looked on in total and complete astonishment.

"Hold on for a moment," I interrupted. "I have no care package in place. I have no adaptions. Mum's bed is two floors up the stairs. She can't climb the stairs."

"Don't worry about that," Dr Harding replied dismissively.

"We can arrange for paramedics to carry your mum up and down the stairs each day."

I simply couldn't believe what she was saying. There was absolutely no way Mum could be discharged that Friday. In any event, I was previously advised the discharge process would be carefully planned and coordinated. I was told Mum would have a maximum care package in place, with carers coming in three times a day, morning, lunch, and evening.

"Your mum is medically fit," Dr Harding retorted angrily. "If your mum stays in longer, she is at risk of infection."

That was the tipping point.

"Please do not use that as a threat," I responded in a calm manner. "No one would want her back home more than me, but there is absolutely no way she can come out without a care package in place. Don't even look at discharging her."

Mum then turned to me and then asked, "Don't you want me home, Mark?"

My heart sank. I knew the junior doctor was playing the emotional game by forcing a wedge between Mum and myself to free up the bed. But I remained calm and resolute.

Dr Harding frowned. She looked incredulous as I was questioning her decision. She left abruptly. Ten minutes later, the senior consultant came round to examine Mum. He was more conciliatory.

After a brief discussion, we agreed that Mum would be discharged on the following Tuesday. That gave me just under a week to sort out our living arrangements at home.

What amazed me, in retrospect, was that the junior doctor was simply oblivious to the care needs of Mum. Her priority was to free up the bed for another patient.

That weekend, I bought a single bed with all the bed clothes. Mum was going to sleep in the living room. I also arranged the delivery of a commode.

7

Our life routine

Discharge from hospital

I remember vividly the day Mum was discharged from the King Edward Hospital. It will stay in my memory forever. I arrived at the ward around mid-afternoon on Tuesday, 16th September 2014.

As part of the discharge process, the pharmacist discussed Mum's medication.

"You need to speak to my son," Mum told her.

Mum needed to take one 15mg mirtazapine tablet at night, for five nights. The pharmacist advised Mum that she also had to take Dalteparin, which is an injected anticoagulant to ensure the thinning of her blood and to stop any blood clotting. "Who will do that?" I questioned the pharmacist.

"You, of course," she pointed out tersely.

"I don't know how to inject a needle into Mum," I argued.

"That's not my problem," the pharmacist replied in a dismissive tone.

Then the pharmacist immediately left Mum and started to walk over to see another patient on the ward.

I just could not believe how she was treating us. I subsequently interrupted her and told her I didn't like her attitude. It was clear she had no appreciation of how to talk to elderly patients. The pharmacist looked at me with a blank expression. I was not going to receive any assistance from her.

I subsequently spoke to the Matron, who apologised. She arranged for a District Nurse to visit Mum every day and administer the injection.

By 2 pm that afternoon, Mum was fully dressed and sitting on her bed. She had been promised that an ambulance would arrive by 3 pm to take her home. I subsequently inquired to see if I could travel with her. Due to insurance reasons, however, I wasn't allowed to travel in the ambulance.

As Mum was sitting on the bed, a nurse walked over to her. The nurse then went to take Mum's Zimmer frame away.

"This is the NHS frame," she hastily remarked to Mum. "You can't take it home."

Once again, I interrupted. Mum's eyes rolled as if to say, *Mark, please not again.*

"Are you being serious? Look at her, she can hardly walk," I asserted. "She is not leaving the hospital without it."

"Just for the record," I added, "two weeks ago, the occupational therapist advised me that Mum could keep it. We are not stealing anything."

The nurse shrugged her shoulders and left, annoyed. She reported me to the Matron. A few hours later the Matron walked over to me and once again apologised.

Home, sweet home

Around 3:30 pm, I decided to go back home and wait for Mum. The hours passed. Six o'clock, seven o'clock, eight o'clock in the evening went by, with no sign of the ambulance or Mum. I phoned the ward nurse. She told me that Mum was still there, sitting on her bed, waiting for the ambulance to arrive.

I informed her that Mum had been waiting since 2 pm. The nurse apologised. I told the nurse that if the ambulance did not pick Mum up in thirty minutes, she would have to stay in the hospital another night. Fifteen minutes later, the nurse rang me back and told me that Mum was in the process of being transferred to the ambulance. Once again, the hours passed. Mum arrived home at 10:30pm in a large taxi. The driver helped Mum out of the vehicle. She thanked him.

She looked very frail and thin. She was determined, however, to walk to her front door unaided, with just her Zimmer frame. As she got to the door, she sighed heavily with relief and pure joy.

There was no fanfare, no coronation—just me, waiting at the door, with the light of the full moon shining on our house. Nevertheless, it was one of the happiest days of my life to see her arrive home.

Mum shuffled through the front door. She paused, took a breath, and then her eyes opened wide in pure wonderment and delight as she had not seen our living room for five and a half weeks. It was so beautiful to see the warmth and joy on her face.

Her single bed was now located at the far end of the living room. Next to it, I put some brightly coloured flowers on the table. Although she didn't particularly like the colour of the duvet cover, she commented that I had made the room look beautiful.

I helped her to sit down on the sofa and made her a cup of tea. Afterwards, I tucked her comfortably into her new bed. That night, she slept soundly.

The next morning, around 6 am, I heard Mum shouting for me. I quickly rushed down the stairs. I walked into the living room. Mum was just in the process of getting up from the bed. She had just soiled all the bedclothes, and there was running diarrhoea on the floor.

She was distraught, agitated, and panicking. She was in a lot of emotional discomfort. She was shaking. I quickly comforted her, saying to her tenderly, "It's okay," and, "Don't worry."

I quickly managed to lift Mum onto the sofa. Then I threw the bed sheets away and started to clean and disinfect the floor. For about ten minutes, Mum was disorientated. Thankfully however, I managed to calm her down.

Mum noticed I had purchased a commode. "I'm not going to use that," she announced with clarity. She told me she would walk to the toilet when she needed it. So we threw it away. After only two weeks of being home, she started to use her walking stick rather than the Zimmer frame. She was fierce in safeguarding her physical independence. And while she got used to her walking stick, she despised all the other aids associated with old age and infirmity.

Daily living

I appreciated the fact that having been a very independent woman (going out shopping each day), to be confined and living in one room, was going to be very difficult for Mum.

A routine of eating, drinking fluids (to maintain hydration throughout the day), and regular exercise was the only way, in my opinion, to improve Mum's quality of life and give her back a level of independence she so desperately missed,

I was always balancing between what she was able to do for herself and what daily activities she required a level of support.

We soon established a daily routine. For me, it was the only way of getting through the day without feeling despondent and disheartened. In many ways, we fell into a comfortable pattern that suited both of us.

So, our typical day proceeded as follows:

Mum would wake up around 6:30 am (during all of her life, she was always an early riser).

Even before I woke up and got down the stairs, Mum managed to dress and make her bed. Personal hygiene and keeping the home clean and immaculate were some of the fundamental core values in her life, and she wasn't going to change because of her illness.

I would then make her breakfast. This would consist of either cereal or porridge. A carer would arrive around 9 am and give Mum a wash. Sometimes it would be a strip wash or just washing her face and back. Around 11 am, we would either have a boiled egg with toast, ham, or a chicken sandwich. That would be followed by dinner at 4 pm, which usually consisted of roast chicken, peas, carrots, or a steak pie. And then, around 6 pm, we would have a dessert, which would typically be apple or rhubarb crumble and ice cream, or perhaps a lemon or strawberry cheesecake.

The day was interspersed with three or four cups of tea with one or two biscuits.

At the end of each day, I would check how many calories Mum had consumed. The dietician recommended about 3,000 calories a day. That was an impossible task for Mum. I was, however, satisfied that Mum was consuming in around 1,800 calories a day.

Also, Mum's doctor prescribed a nutritional supplement drink designed for cancer patients. It contained around 350 calories and 13 grams of protein. Initially, Mum refused to drink them.

I kept urging and cajoling Mum to drink at least three bottles a day, but I soon gathered that the more I pushed, the more Mum refused to entertain the idea of drinking even one bottle. "If it is so good, you taste it," she would often say to me. So I did. And she was right. It tasted vile. I reminded her that it wasn't the taste that was important, but the nutrition it gave her. That argument didn't wash with Mum.

It soon became apparent that, while she wouldn't listen to me, she would take notice of the carer who came in the morning to wash her. Encouraged by the carer, Mum reluctantly started to consume one nutrition drink a day.

As a result of our daily routine, together with the exercise programme I put in place, Mum's weight gain over the next six months was impressive and remarkable. I would weigh Mum every week. She so desperately wanted to put on weight.

From weighing only six stone when she came out of the hospital in September 2014, Mum reached seven stone ten pounds in January 2015. She then gained more weight, where she reached eight stone four pounds by March 2015. Not only did her weight increase, but her mobility also significantly improved. I felt comfortable leaving her alone for a few hours each day.

Mum was progressing well, so much so that it was my intention to go back to work.

I arranged for carers to come in three times a day, morning, lunch time, and early afternoon, to attend to Mum. At this stage, Mum was capable of going into the kitchen by herself and boiling an egg or making a sandwich for lunch. The carers were skilled, dedicated, and compassionate, which gave me the extra reassurance I needed that Mum would be looked after during the day.

With the care provision in place, and with my 12 weeks of unpaid leave at work coming to the end very quickly, my employer and I devised a return to work plan, with reduced hours for the first two weeks and then going back full time after that.

On my first day back, I discovered that my role and responsibilities, in fact my entire function, had been transferred. My employer arbitrarily sidelined and demoted me to more demeaning activities. In effect, I had no job.

My employer wilfully breached my employment contract. Their motive was clear: to oust me from the organisation. It also wasn't surprising to me, as I was aware many months ago that they wanted to remove me. I was simply unlucky. I was in the wrong place, at the wrong time, with the wrong people around me. I joined a toxic, pernicious and dysfunctional working environment. I take, however, full responsibility for allowing myself to get into such a situation. I should have seen the warning signs and arranged my exit from the company much sooner. What did surprise me, however, was their sheer callousness and ruthlessness. I saw with my own eyes, bigotry and hatefulness, which I hope I will never see again in my lifetime.

During the first week back at work, my self-esteem and self-worth crumbled, and I felt completely overwhelmed. Night after night, I would wake up in the early hours and felt gripped and terrorised with anxiety and fear. I began feeling tired and sad and was quickly heading into a downward spiral. I doubted my abilities. I doubted who I was. I questioned my self-worth. I doubted my very own existence. Most of all, I questioned my faith. I covered up all of this for Mum. I knew that I could not show her what I was going through.

For two solid weeks, I started to gamble and lose heavily in order to numb out all the pain. I was in the process of throwing my life away. In short, I was heading for a downward spiral of self-destruction. With such an addiction, I first had to recognise I had a problem. As I was in denial, this was not easy. With all addictions (gambling is no exception), I had to work out how to deal with the problem. I had two choices facing me. Either, I tried to avoid the 'triggers' that made me want to gamble in the first place. Or, I simply abstained from the gambling addiction. Thankfully, I chose the latter. A voice inside myself told me to stop. And I did. I pulled myself back from the dark place I did not want to go.

I remember one evening, I was lying in bed, thinking to myself that I simply couldn't handle all of this. I felt emotionally paralysed. I knew, however, that if I disintegrated and entered the dark place of my depression, I would bring my Mum down too, as she was entirely reliant on me, physically, emotionally, and financially. It is not an understatement to say that her sheer survival was relying on me. I had a choice to make. Do I just give up and go into my own downward spiral of despair? Or do I carry on? It was then that I prayed for strength.

During a restless and sleepless night, I turned on the radio for some comfort. I just happened to catch a song called *Last Minute* by an artist called Josephine. The chorus line resonated and spoke deep within my heart.

The next morning, as I woke up, I knew my prayers had been answered. I found my inner strength. The only thing that mattered in my life was not to let Mum down.

As for work, I knew I deserved better than to be treated in that manner. So the next day, I took back control of the situation. And more importantly, I took back control of my life. I immediately resigned. It was all but in name, constructive dismissal. I remembered the advice Mum gave me when I was young: "Do unto others as you would have them do unto you." I was determined my peace of mind would not be destroyed. One of my closest friends gave me some profound advice. "No one can take any power away from you because they never gave it to you in the first place. Don't you see Mark, it is not theirs to take. The power lies within you and no one else. Don't forget who you are. Your Mum has strength of character. And so do you. Search for your inner ego strength."

On my last day at work, I prayed. And from somewhere, I found a space within my heart to forgive my employer. Forgiveness was paramount to my emotional and inner healing, as the alternative was to allow bitterness and resentment of the injustice to fester within me all my life. I was determined not to live my life full of hatefulness but instead one of peace and harmony.

I remember the famous Holocaust survivor, Viktor E. Frankl, once said that, "Everything can be taken from a man but one thing: the last of the human freedoms—to choose one's attitude in any given set of circumstances, to choose one's own way." So I chose to forgive my employer.

I walked out the door with dignity and peace within my heart and never looked back. I went home that evening and once again looked at my charter.

I chose not to tell Mum what had happened that day at work, as I knew she would start worrying about me. That was the last thing I wanted her to do. So the following week, I left home at the same time in the mornings. Mum believed I was going to work. Instead, the harsh reality was that I was walking the streets of London, looking for work.

After a week, I told Mum that my employer had given me some more time off. I was uncomfortable telling her a half-truth. But to paraphrase Marlon Brando, the famous American actor, "Everyone lies. We lie for peace; we lie for tranquillity; we lie for love." I freely admit I lied to Mum out of love. To protect her from worrying and not to cause her any unnecessary distress.

Two weeks after I resigned from my job, I found a part-time role. It was ideal for me, as it was three days a week. For the other two days, I could be at home looking after Mum. I knew somewhere a guardian angel was watching over me.

Fighting spirit

In October 2014, a young community physiotherapist started to come round every week to see Mum. He started showing Mum a few exercises to improve her mobility. Mum was reluctant at first, but eventually decided to do them.

It was clear from the start that he was not used to dealing with an alert, lucid, and coherent elderly person. I kept repeating to him that Mum was fiercely independent, but he refused to listen. While he was helpful and encouraging, he would challenge Mum. However, Mum was not a person to be challenged and, therefore, a clash was inevitable. On one occasion, the physiotherapist arrived with a bath seat for Mum to sit on when she takes her next shower. He wanted Mum to try it out. He insisted that Mum needed to walk up the flight of stairs to the bathroom.

Mum was insistent she did not want to walk upstairs. At first, she quietly refused. The physiotherapist was persistent. After about thirty minutes of arguing, Mum reluctantly agreed. The physiotherapist and I supported Mum up the twenty steps.

Once in the bathroom, the altercation occurred.

"I want you to sit on the seat," the physiotherapist announced firmly.

"I am not going to use it," Mum replied. "I am not going to sit on it."

Three times he insisted that she should try to sit on the seat, which straddled each side of the bath.

On the fourth time of asking Mum to sit on the board, his attitude became condescending.

Mum then exploded with anger.

"You are not listening to me. I have told you four times; I don't want to sit on the board," Mum said angrily. "I may have cancer but my mind is still there. I am not dead yet. I know what you are talking about, and I simply do not want to use the bath board."

I saw his bulging veins in the back of his neck.

He then pointed out sarcastically, "I am only doing my job, darling."

"Don't call me darling," Mum responded.

I just stood there watching them. I decided not to intervene as I could see Mum was more than capable of handling the situation. As both of them were locked in this argument, I suddenly burst out into laughter. They turned their heads in unison and looked at me in astonishment.

I laughed because I could see the fight and spirit within Mum. She still had that determination, tenacity, and resilience.

The physiotherapist left quickly. He never returned. Mum could not believe his attitude.

"Because I'm old and hard of hearing, it doesn't mean my mind has gone," she added. "It was as if as though he was talking down and belittling me just because I'm old. I'm not going to be treated like that." She was furious.

8

Looking forward to Christmas 2014

With the physiotherapist refusing to visit Mum again, I knew it was crucial to improve her muscle and bone strength.

About three weeks before Christmas, I bought some exercise resistance bands. Fortunately, a few years previously, I had employed a personal trainer. He was fantastic as he showed me how to exercise safely, which allowed me to deploy those same exercises with Mum.

Mum and I soon established an exercise routine. In the mornings, around 10:30 am, I would sit on Mum's bed and show her how to use the lightweight resistance bands.

"I've done it. Now you can do it," I would say. And to her credit, she did. She was enthusiastic. When she achieved eight reps, I would encourage her further. "Just another two reps," I would say.

I started to set out an exercise programme for her, recording the number of reps she would do each time. We would exercise every other day, focusing on the upper body in the first session and the lower body the next. I taught her to do squats, heel raises, toe raises, triceps curls, upper back exercises, knee extension exercises, and overhead chest presses, all with the resistance bands.

In addition to these activities, of her free will, Mum would walk around the living room and hallway with her walking stick for about five minutes. I even bought her a digital stepometer, and we counted how many steps she walked each day. Jokingly, Mum commented she was training for a marathon race. We both laughed.

As well as establishing a physical exercise regime, I had to also ensure Mum was psychologically healthy. I remember reading many years ago, that both nostalgia and reminiscing reduced anxiety. I would, therefore, encourage Mum to talk about her memories of the past, especially when she was a child during the wartime Blitz.

I kept Mum mentally active so her mind was sharp and alert. Every other day, we would sit down next to each other on the sofa. We would play some memory game applications on my iPad. We had a lot of fun. In particular, I chose games that would stimulate her frontal cortex in order to improve her short-term memory, the speed in which she processed information and her problem solving skills. In one specific game that Mum played, she had to remember different sets of animal picture sequences. By playing this game over a two-month period, Mum reached level seventeen out of a total of twenty-four levels. She was very pleased with herself. I played the game alongside her, and I could only reach level ten. I was pleased that her mind was sharp and her short-term memory was good.

In many ways, Mum's quality of life was improving.

Christmas shopping

Over the previous months, I would take Mum out for short walks. Because of Mum's frailty, she only managed to walk to the top of our road and back, about a five-minute walk.

Mum was determined to do the Christmas shopping, as she had done in all previous years. So in the middle of December 2014, we decided to go out to the shops in the high street. I was by her side. She hung on to me. She walked a whole mile to the shops.

We arrived at the supermarket, which she hadn't seen for

over seven months. As we entered the door to the supermarket, Mum was looking down at the pavement. Then she looked up. Her little eyes lit up and opened widely. Her whole face glowed. Her smile was so large. It covered up all the wrinkles on her face.

She was like a small child walking into Disneyland for the very first time. To see the pure, innocent, and magical joy on her face was profoundly beautiful and humbling to witness and something I will never forget.

We walked up and down each of the aisles within the supermarket. Mum loved every second that passed. She looked out for any of her friends, whom not so long ago she would have met shopping. Sadly, she didn't see any of them.

After spending thirty minutes in there, grasping on to each other, with Mum unsteady on her feet, she walked out of there with her eyes still open with pure wonder. We then managed to walk home. That day she amazed me. Through sheer determination, she walked two miles.

That night, I tucked her into bed. She was overwhelmed with joyful emotion.

Christmas Dinner

It was Christmas Day.

Mum was determined that Christmas Day would be no different from our beautiful Christmases we had had in years before. I think Mum knew this was going to be our final Christmas Day spent together.

As I was about to cook the Christmas dinner, Mum shuffled into the kitchen. "I'm going to cook the meal," she said with a soft, loving tone. "Just go and relax."

I hovered outside the kitchen, watching Mum cook the meal just in case she got into any difficulties. There was no need. She knew precisely what she was doing.

As the Christmas dinner was cooking, Mum also laid

out the table with cutlery, napkins, glasses, and so on. I could only watch in wonder at her sheer resilience and determination.

Mum's sister, Jenny, bought her a fleeced, turquoise pyjamas as a Christmas present. She wore them that night. She looked so warm and comfortable in them.

"They are lovely," she kept saying to me. "I don't want to spoil them as they are so nice."

Christmas Day was over in a blink of an eye. She had only vomited once. We had an excellent Christmas meal and a peaceful day. That was all I could have hoped for.

9

Entering the final journey, 2015

In January 2015, Mum had a further CT scan.

In February 2015, we saw Dr Barlow, the clinical oncologist, at the King Edward Hospital. The appointment was to discuss the results of January's scan. On the day, we waited over two hours in the reception area before we were shown into Dr Barlow's room.

Dr Barlow turned round in her chair."I have to apologise, but your scan results haven't arrived yet. Don't worry, I have some other images from before, and they look fine. You are doing well," she said to Mum in a cheerful and relaxed way. "I will chase up the results. I suggest you have a blood test now, and I will call your son on his mobile phone about the results. Come back in six months' time for your next appointment."

After only five minutes, we were led out of the room.

I felt a sense of relief.

"This is great news," I declared to Mum joyfully.

Mum was quiet. She was not so sure. She knew Dr Barlow had got it wrong. She was right. It was the calm before the storm.

Thirty minutes later, as Mum was having her blood test, my mobile phone rang. It was Dr Barlow.

"I'm afraid I have some bad news for you," she advised. "I regret to say the results of the scan have confirmed our worst fears. There are two spots near the lymph nodes. You need to make an appointment in one month."

"Hold on for a moment," I replied, shocked. "Just 30 minutes ago you stated everything was okay."

"I know. I'm so sorry," she admitted hesitantly. Then she put the phone down. The conversation lasted only a few seconds.

The news penetrated my emotions' defences. I then had to walk back into the medical room where Mum was sitting, having her blood test and of course, tell her the news. It was a dreadful experience. I was stricken. I stood frozen in the doorway.

Mum paused and took a deep breath.

"Tell me straight," Mum said taking a further deep breath. "Tell me everything. I knew there was something wrong."

I felt a lump in my throat. I looked at her in silence. The words I wanted to say were stuck. I could not speak.

"I knew it," Mum said in a soft, tender, but overwhelming sad voice.

After a deep breath, I simply repeated what Dr Barlow told me. I did not hold anything back.

We came back home. We were now in complete limbo. We had to wait a further four weeks to find out the true extent of the spots they found.

Being told

In March 2015, we went back to the King Edward Hospital to see Dr Barlow. But instead, we saw a junior registrar.

We were shown into a small room. The registrar was young. As we entered the room, the registrar was nervously twisting her fingers. Rather than looking Mum in the eyes, the registrar looked constantly down to the floor as she was speaking to Mum, interspersed with slight glimpses in Mum's eyes.

"Do you want a blunt conversation?" she enquired.

"Yes," Mum replied bravely and without any hesitation in her voice.

"You have some microscopic cells that have invaded the tissues around your right colon and lymph nodes. These cells will become a mass. Without palliative chemotherapy treatment, you are looking at months. With chemotherapy treatment, which has only one in four chance of helping you, you may last possibly a year. The side effects of the chemotherapy, however, in your case would be severe. At the moment, I believe you are still far too weak to have chemotherapy."

From the hospital's point of view, Mum's best interest was to let nature take its own course. Looking at Mum's frailty, it was the most humanitarian and caring decision to make. One that I agreed with.

At the end of the conversation, Mum said respectfully and calmly to the registrar, "Thank you so very much. Thank you for all your help." Mum said it in such a way that it seemed like she were saying it to a cashier at a supermarket helping her to pack her shopping bags.

The registrar looked startled at how well Mum took the news. "Do you understand what I have just said?" the registrar repeated to Mum.

With immense clarity, Mum nodded. While Mum didn't know what palliative care meant, she fully understood what the registrar was saying to her.

As we arrived back home that day, Mum conceded she had no hope. I told her that we always have hope. I knew, however, Mum's decline was inevitable. As her son, I was now entering the most stressful period of my entire life.

Palliative care support was virtually non-existent. A Macmillan nurse was assigned to Mum. He initially started to come around to see Mum once a week, but then he suddenly stopped. I was unable to contact him. He was always on holiday. I complained but all to no avail.

Disturbingly, Mum was not receiving any meaningful treatment or advice on pain control from the Macmillan nurse. He explained the only effective pain control was to stop the pain in the first place. This could only be achieved if Mum was heavily sedated throughout the day, he advised.

Without any palliative care, I had to constantly ring Mum's doctor. She always had time for Mum. She was wonderful.

During her visits, she would determine the most effective pain control for Mum. Although, there was very little she could do given the advanced state of Mum's cancer. For the majority of the time, Mum would take up to eight paracetamols a day.

On one particular home visit by the doctor, the issue of cardiopulmonary resuscitation was approached. Because of Mum being hard of hearing, she did not understand what the doctor was saying to her. The doctor subsequently asked me to explain to Mum. It was a difficult and sensitive conversation.

I took a deep breath and, in a calm voice, I explained, "Mum if you have a heart attack, the doctors in the hospital will just allow things to take their natural course." She looked at me and nodded. She understood. In front of the doctor, Mum agreed, if the event occurred, she would not be resuscitated. I believe that was the right decision, as I knew that only five percent of resuscitations on the elderly were successful. Mum just wanted to be allowed to die naturally.

Three weeks after seeing the doctor, Mum began to feel increasingly nauseous. It came on without warning. Each night, I would put Mum to bed and leave my bedroom door open listening out for any noise, hoping she was sleeping okay. She would have a glass of water on a table and a bucket next to her bed.

Every night, Mum would feel sick. As soon as I heard a noise, I would immediately rush down the stairs.

As I ran into the living room, Mum would be vomiting uncontrollably into the bucket.

I would ensure she was sitting upright with her head forward facing into the bucket. I would comfort and reassure her, saying, "It's okay. It's alright. I'm here." As Mum was vomiting, her right hand would shake uncontrollably to such an extent she was incapable of holding the glass of water. I would, therefore, hold the glass up to her mouth as she would take a few tiny sips.

After about five to ten minutes, Mum would stop vomiting and feel better. I would make her comfortable and tuck her into bed again. It was one of the most distressing sights to witness Mum in such a vulnerable state. Tears would be streaming down my face as I comforted her. I felt so helpless and so powerless. After she had finished vomiting, I would make sure she was settled in bed. I would then wash and disinfect the bucket. Every night, I would lay awake, my door open, worrying if Mum would choke on her own vomit during the night.

Mum's doctor prescribed a range of anti-sickness tablets,- none of which had any real effect. During the day, Mum would eat her meal. About ten minutes later, she would vomit the whole meal back up again. Mum was nearing the end of her life. It was clearly evident that Mum could not be left on her own and needed 24-hour nursing care. I immediately gave up my three-day-a-week job to look after her full time.

Final direction

In April 2015, we returned to the King Edward Hospital. Once again, we saw the clinical oncologist, Dr Barlow.

"You look very frail," she claimed as she stared at Mum.

Mum asked how long she had to live.

"Well, most cases such as yours, patients do not survive beyond six months after their operation," Dr Barlow cited. "You are in your seventh month now, so you are doing well."

Mum looked devastated. "Are you saying I should have died by now?"

Dr Barlow sighed. She totally ignored Mum's question. "We will discharge you. There is no need to come back anymore. The palliative care team will take responsibility for you."

Then without warning, Dr Barlow simply got up and hurried away out of the room, never to be seen again. She didn't even say goodbye. She completely ignored Mum. Mum looked at me, her eyes wide and sad. They looked watery. It was as if Dr Barlow discarded Mum like rubbish on a litter-strewn wasteland.

A young nurse was left in the room. She asked Mum whether she had booked herself into a hospice.

I pointed out that it was not a luxury hotel. She giggled.

I knew I had to get Mum out of that room and out of the hospital quickly.

Mum was devastated. She left the room a broken shell.

I could not believe the complete lack of sensitivity and the unprofessional approach by Dr Barlow. The way Mum was treated was appalling and horrendous. No one should be treated like that, let alone my Mum.

Mum forbade me to complain on her behalf. In many respects, that was the worst weekend of my life. A veil of sadness came over everything in my life as I watched the Mum I loved slowly change. She looked physically and emotionally drained. She disintegrated in front of my very eyes. Dr Barlow took away all hope. Mum had simply given up, as her worst fear had come true. Death was no longer in the distance. It was imminent. She was now looking death straight in the face.

Once again, I was rendered helpless. I had no answers. I was infuriated with the way Dr Barlow behaved toward Mum. I had to make a choice once again. Do I complain, which would not change Mum's situation and would use up all my energy, or do I let the event pass over me?

During the weekend, I read my charter again. As at so many other times, it was my cornerstone. I also continued to pray.

Then, as the shock of being told in such a callous and uncaring nature wore away, Mum started to show some fight again. She managed somehow to emerge from her darkness. Her indomitable, tenacious human spirit reappeared.

"I've had a good life. I suppose I can't complain. I've reached 80 years old. My luck has just run out," she said to me. "When your time is up, it is up and there is nothing you can do about it." She still felt intensely alive.

"If you can help me with the stairs to my bedroom, I can

sort out my belongings. I know it will be tough for you to sort them out when I've gone," she said to me.

"Don't worry about that," I replied.

"Mark, you need to be strong about this," she added. I could see she was deeply worried about me.

Over Sunday dinner, Mum asked me to bring in her shopping bag that was hanging up in the hallway. I gave it to her. She opened her bag and pulled out her purse. She said, "There is two hundred and fifty pounds cash for you." I just managed to hold back my tears. "It took me a year to save it," she added. It was her life's savings. I told her that I would buy a tie and put the rest in a bank account.

Two weeks of pain management

Family and friends used to say I was strong. If only they knew. I didn't feel strong a

lot of the time. It was a matter of simply getting through each day. On occasions, Mum would squeeze my hand gently as a way of encouragement. She knew watching her die was tough for me.

Mum's health started its inevitable decline. By now, Mum was mostly expressing her pain not so much in agitation, but by grimacing. She desperately tried to conceal it, but by this stage, it was far too intense.

My nerves and body would twitch like a rabbit if Mum looked in any kind of discomfort. I would constantly ask her how she felt. Worrying about Mum 24 hours a day was emotionally and physically draining.

Naive as it may sound, more than anything in the world, I wanted her pain to vanish.

During the day, Mum would be sitting on the sofa watching television. On occasions, I would be laying on top of her bed in the sitting room, with my headphones on. I had given her all my love but sadly, love was not enough to save her from the pain. She didn't know it but I was actually praying for her. Prayer was now all I had left. So I prayed that I had enough strength for both of us. I prayed that God spared her the pain of the cancer and gave it to me instead.

Our lives were now in limbo. We both knew her health would decline. But what we didn't know was when and how the decline will happen. Simply waiting for her to deteriorate was heart-breaking. Every morning, I looked at my charter. I repeated to myself, take one day at a time.

As Mum's grimacing became more and more acute, it was time to increase the pain relief medication. So to ease her suffering, Mum was now on what is commonly called in the medical profession opioid analgesics. In short, strong painkilling drugs.

At first, the Macmillan nurse recommended BuTrans patches. These patches contained the ingredient buprenorphine. This drug is related to morphine.

As I didn't know where to place the patch, I asked the Macmillan nurse to place the patch on Mum for me. He refused as it wasn't his job. I subsequently rang for a District Nurse to show me. Because they were short of staff, they were reluctant to visit Mum. But after I complained, they agreed to visit.

That afternoon, I received a ring at the door. It was a District Nurse. As it so happened, she arrived at the door at the very same time Mum began to violently vomit.

I rushed to the door and let her in the house. I then immediately ran back into the living room to comfort Mum. The District Nurse walked in the living room and sat down on a chair.

"Well, where is the patch?" she quipped in an annoying tone of voice.

She could see Mum was vomiting and in distress.

"Hold on, surely you can see Mum is being sick," I replied.

The District Nurse remained silent. I could see she was annoyed visiting Mum. She did not have one ounce of empathy. Thankfully, Mum was oblivious to her attitude.

After I managed to get Mum settled, the District Nurse showed me how to place the patch on Mum. Then the District Nurse immediately left.

Mum's doctor prescribed further controlled drugs that I needed to administer. I was extremely apprehensive, as any overdose could have been lethal. I recorded Mum's medication every day.

She had eight paracetamols spread throughout the day, OxyNorm (which I injected into her mouth) morning and at night, and Levorphanol, which I gave her twice a day.

These drugs would ensure Mum was not in any pain, but at the same time, were destroying her quality of life. Mum was sedated and completely unconscious for most of the day. As I watched her sleep, I was once again rendered helpless. I would pray to the heavens to look over her. To protect her. To be her blanket as she softly slept. She would wake up in small bursts. It was heartrending to watch her in this state.

The choice that faced me as a carer and as Mum's son was twofold. Do I stop administering these controlled drugs to Mum, and as a consequence she would spend the whole day in pain? Or alternatively, do I administer her the drugs to ease her pain, but as a result, she would be heavily sedated throughout the day?

I literally had Mum's quality of life in my hands each day.

Watching her like this, I was convinced she urgently needed 24-hour medical care, which I was unable to provide at home.

10

Mum's final days

Turning point of mum's illness

I will never forget Saturday, 19 April 2015. It marked a pivotal point in Mum's illness.

That morning, as usual, Mum woke up and made her bed. But on this occasion, she seemed very different.

"I simply can't do it," she commented exhaustively.

"That's fine," I replied, trying to comfort her.

"I feel so unwell," she kept repeating. I could see her grimacing throughout the morning.

She refused to see the doctor. Then, at 10:30 am, she started vomiting. As the day progressed, she vomited about six times. She still, however, refused to see the doctor. Around 7 pm that night, I tucked her into bed. About an hour later, I heard a loud bump. I immediately rushed down the stairs. I saw Mum there, sitting on the floor, vomiting uncontrollably in the bucket, with diarrhoea all over the floor. She was completely disorientated.

I immediately lifted her up gently onto the sofa. I comforted her, cleaned her up, and cleaned and disinfected the floor. There was absolutely no way she could carry on like this without receiving medical attention.

I didn't know what to do, so I rang for the ambulance around 8:30 pm.

Two hours passed. There was no sign of the ambulance. I

subsequently rang again to find out what was going on. They apologised and advised they would send out a crew again.

The ambulance finally arrived at 12:30 am, a good four hours after I originally contacted them.

The paramedic walked into our living room, looked at Mum and then started to question me as to the reason why I phoned for emergency services.

"She needs urgent medical attention," I replied.

"Well they don't like taking in these sort of cases in the Accident and Emergency Department, it skews their targets," he moaned. "You should have called the out-of-hours doctor instead."

"Are you serious? Look at the state of her," I replied in total disbelief. Mum kept on insisting that she was fine.

Eventually, the paramedic agreed to take her in the ambulance. We arrived in Accident and Emergency Department at St John's Hospital at 12:45 am.

Upon arrival, Mum was wheeled into a small cubicle room. The room was freezing. I subsequently complained. I was advised that the air conditioning couldn't be turned off. The nurses gave Mum two extra blankets. I also put my jacket over her. We waited a further four hours to see a consultant doctor.

"We were waiting for a bed in a ward for your Mum," he announced.

It was now about 5 am. I was completely shattered. Mum wanted me to go home. The doctor advised me she would be okay, and there was no need for me to stay.

Reluctantly, I left Mum and headed home and went straight to bed. I had about four hours of sleep.

I arrived back at the hospital around 2 pm the next day. The woman on the main

reception desk apologised because the computer system had crashed the night before, and she had no record of my mother being admitted to the hospital.

"You can't have lost my Mum," I concurred. "Are you telling me you are totally reliant on the computer system?"

She nodded.

The receptionist phoned around to a number of different wards, all to no avail. She asked me to check with five separate departments; again, all to no avail. Then, after two hours of searching, the receptionist discovered that, in fact, Mum hadn't been moved from the small cubicle room in the Accident and Emergency Department she was in the night before. I immediately rushed over to see her.

I found her cold, shaking, and shivering.

"Mark, please don't complain," Mum insisted.

I immediately saw the nurse in charge. The nurse apologised and admitted they simply could not find a bed on the ward. I immediately asked that they put a portable heater in the room. I told them that I was not leaving until they found a bed for her.

Two hours later, she was transferred to a general medical ward.

Admitted to hospital

On Monday morning, another oncologist consultant came round to see Mum. Thankfully, I was present.

"Do you know what is going on, Mrs Carrington?" he asked softly.

"I have a few cells that are cancerous," she replied.

"Yes, that's right. But there are sadly more than just a few," he confirmed in a soft and warm tone. "We can't treat them. We will make you comfortable."

"Thank you so much," Mum replied.

I sat with Mum all day.

At 7:30 pm that evening, a palliative nurse took me aside and informed me gently that it would be unlikely that Mum would survive beyond the weekend.

"It's time to prepare yourself," she concluded.

It was a total shock. As she delivered the devastating news, she could see my inner struggle not to burst out crying. But I could not hold back. Without warning, I erupted into a flood of tears. They came from a hidden place deep within me.

Once I gathered my thoughts, I began to tell her about Mum's life. Our conversation lasted over two hours. That evening, I just couldn't face going home so, instead, I stayed in a local hotel for the night.

Mum seemed oblivious to what was going on and how close to death she was. The palliative nurse was so kind and gentle towards Mum.

During the entire weekend, the hospital provided only a skeleton service of medical cover.

On Sunday evening, I noticed that the syringe driver that was dispensing morphine into Mum was empty. Mum was in agony, but once again would not complain. So I called the nurse over to the bed and explained that the driver needed replacing.

"What do you want me to do?" she asked.

"You are the nurse. You should know," I replied.

The nurse pondered. "I don't know how to administer the morphine through the driver. I haven't had any training in this field. I will need to call a consultant," she admitted.

It was clear to me that the nurse had insufficient training and had no idea of how to care for a person dying.

We then had to wait for an hour until the consultant arrived to change the syringe driver.

I did not want Mum to pass away in hospital. Statistically, around 500,000 people die in the UK each year. Just over fifty three per cent will die in a hospital. I was determined for Mum not to be one of them. She deserved to pass away in a hospice, where she could be given compassionate care and spend her final moments in peace and dignity.

As Mum was on a general medical ward, there were all different women there. In the bed adjacent to Mum was a young woman, probably no more than 20 years old. She kept playing her radio loudly. One time she was singing along to the song *Girls Just Want to Have Fun* by Cyndi Lauper. The young woman was not to know how seriously ill Mum was at the time, but it simply didn't seem right. Mum should have never have been on this ward.

"Mum deserves better than this. She is not going to be shunned away in a hospital ward surrounded by young women playing music as she is laying there dying," I insisted firmly to the ward nurse.

The ward nurse and I both agreed that the hospital ward Mum was on was totally inappropriate.

Thankfully, Mum survived the weekend. On the following day, I demanded that Mum be moved to a hospice. I was advised there were no beds available in any of the local hospices.

Then on Tuesday, arrangements were being made to transfer her to a hospice on the other side of London, approximately fifty miles away from me.

I complained. About five hours later, I was advised that a bed had been found in a hospice local to me, only two miles away.

Hospice care

After successfully arguing Mum's case, on Wednesday morning, Mum was transferred to a local hospice.

The consultant advised me that because Mum was so gravely ill, she could pass away in the ambulance travelling on the way there. I fully understood the risks involved, but she needed to get out of the hospital.

As I was leaving, I hugged the nurse.

She looked at me with tears running down her face.

"Mark, the hospice will take care of your mum now," she said sympathetically. "You have done fantastically, but as your Mum is reaching her final moments, you can now be her son and not her carer."

That afternoon, I went home and prayed as Mum was travelling in the ambulance to the hospice.

I arrived at the hospice around 3:30 pm that day. It was a

wonderful place. Full of light. It had 13 beds for inpatients. Mum had her own room, en-suite bathroom, and television. As I walked into her room, she looked calm and serene. She was lying in bed, propped up by brilliant white pillows. She had her glasses on and was watching her favourite television programme.

I was only with her for less than five minutes when suddenly one of the doctors beckoned me. "I need to talk to you," she ordered.

I left Mum and walked into a small waiting room. As I sat down, I suddenly burst into tears. It was the shock of seeing Mum finally in the hospice. I knew this was now the final chapter.

Naturally, I thought the doctor was going to explain how the hospice will be caring for Mum.

"I want to raise an issue with you," she pointed out sternly.

"Okay," I replied.

"This hospice is for short stay patients only. For up to two weeks. If your mum survives more than our target date, she will either need to go home or go into a care home."

I simply could not believe what I was hearing. Through my blurring eyes, I looked at her and in disbelief replied, "Have you seen my Mum? Have you examined her? She is in no fit state to be moved anywhere."

In my conciliatory mode, I advised the doctor that if Mum's health improves, we would cross that bridge when we came to it.

In the back of my mind, I knew there was absolutely no way Mum was going to be moved. If there was one certainty, Mum was going to end her life here at the hospice.

The hospice was open 24 hours a day. This allowed me to come and go when I liked. I felt so privileged to be so close to her every hour of the day.

I would pop in first thing in the morning to see her. I would only stay for about half an hour.

I would return home to do the household chores and go

back to the hospice early in the afternoon. When I was with Mum, most of the time we didn't chat. Once again, my presence was enough. Mum would either be watching television or sleeping.

For the first week or so, Mum was quite content with herself. At times, she would smile and laugh. She felt comfortable in the hospice. Some days, I would walk in the room, and Mum would be asleep. I would sit in the chair next to her. I would sit in peaceful silence waiting for her to awake.

Every day I visited her, I wore a bright red jacket. I would purposely place it on the back of the chair directly in her line of sight. I knew when she woke up, the first thing she would see was my jacket. I wanted to give her the comfort of knowing that I was there with her.

A few more days passed, and Mum was continuing to do well. The nurses, medical and ancillary staff were simply fantastic and amazing. The gentle and compassionate care and attention Mum received was world-class. I couldn't praise them highly enough.

Mum's final decision

I remember vividly, early on Thursday morning, I arrived at the hospice.

Mum noticed I had my hair cut. Short back and sides. She smiled from ear to ear. She was so pleased I was taking care of myself. That morning, Mum was determined to walk to the toilet. She refused to use the walking frame. Instead, she used her walking stick.

As she arrived to the bathroom, she hit the wall with her fists out of pure frustration towards her own frailty. I could see she was still fighting. I watched her in pure admiration as she still had fire in her heart even at this late stage of her illness.

That day, around mid-morning, a team of doctors examined Mum. The senior consultant, Dr Stevens, checked

Mum's pulse. He commented that it was beating slowly and was very weak. He then walked out the room, leaving both mum and myself together. It was clear that she had very little time left.

After two hours, Dr Stevens came back into the room. I was sitting next to Mum.

He pulled up a chair and leaned over towards Mum.

"I wish to talk to you, Marian," he said gently.

With both of his hands, he held Mum's right hand gently. She was looking directly into his eyes. He went on to explain, in a soft voice, that she had two options.

"We can put tubes in you, and you may live a little longer. Or, we can make you comfortable," he said softly. "What would you prefer?"

Mum knew the consequences of what he was saying to her.

Her eyes were as wide open as they could be. As he finished his last words, Mum turned to me and asked what I thought. At which point, I just completely broke uncontrollably down in a flood of tears. Dr Stevens shuffled up closer. He immediately put his arm around me. He knew instinctively, I had to be held as Mum was now tightly gripping my hand.

It was an act of pure grace, kindness and compassion. The depth of which I had never felt before. He showed me mercy when I most needed it.

Then in a spontaneous and beautiful loving moment, with her right hand, Mum reached to a table next to her bed and pulled out a tissue out of the box and gave it to me. Mum wasn't crying. I then turned round and looked at Dr Stevens and he was in tears.

Even when she was told the news, deep in her heart she was still thinking of me and not herself. As the tears were streaming down my face, I laughed as I was the one who was a complete nervous wreck. Mum was serene, peaceful and calm.

"Will I know anything about it?" she asked Dr Stevens with calmness in her voice.

"You will be at peace," he replied. "We will make you comfortable."

Then Mum said with luminous clarity, the most profound words in the most profound moment.

"I wish to be made comfortable," looking directly in Dr Stevens' eyes.

By saying those six words to him, she paradoxically took control of her life by taking control of her own death.

Looking death in the eye, she wanted to die on her own terms.

The conversation lasted less than a minute, but as long as I live, I will never forget it.

She then asked to see her closest sister, Jenny.

That night, before I left the hospice, Mum asked me to sing her a lullaby.

I did. And as I finished, she fell asleep. She looked so much at peace.

At that point in time, the Liverpool Care Pathway was still being implemented. The thought of Mum starving to death was one of the most difficult emotional things I ever had to watch. It was clearly evident that her body was shutting down and could not absorb any food, and therefore feeding her would only prolong her agony.

Dr Stevens honoured his word. Whilst not dying was not an option, he made Mum comfortable, restful, and calm in preparation of her peaceful passing.

The next morning, I visited Mum again. I walked in her room. She was still. Her eyes were closed. She was in a semi-comatose state. I saw her nose running. I wiped it clean. The tissues in the hospice had an rough texture. Thankfully, before I arrived at the hospice, I bought some ultra soft tissues. I used these tissues so her nose didn't feel so sore.

I started to talk to her. Then her hand moved towards me. I sat on the bed while she was lying there. She felt my fingers and then she begun to pull them towards and into her mouth. She then started to suck my thumb. At this stage, I completely broke down in a shower of tears. Then, out of nowhere, I felt a piercing pain in my heart. I then realised that she needed her lips moistened.

I called the nurse, and she supplied a very small tray of water and some toothette swabs – small sponges on the end of sticks. I would dampen her lips. Mum enjoyed that.

11

Saying goodbye

Final weekend

Close family came round and visited Mum during the weekend. Her brothers and sisters said their goodbyes to her. She managed to tell them that she loved them.

Another beautiful and tender moment that will be with me until the day I die, was when Jenny saw Mum lying in her bed at the hospice.

Jenny decided to wear an emerald crystal pendant that Mum had bought her as a present over 50 years before. It had no monetary value, but its sentimental value was priceless.

It happened to be a beautiful summer's day. Jenny was standing near the window in Mum's room when suddenly, out of nowhere, the pendant caught Mum's eye. As the weather was glorious that day, Mum could see it sparkling and glittering as the sun shone on it through the window.

Mum then took a deep breath and gathered all her strength. Her arm was too heavy for her frail bones to hold up. But she managed to raise her hand and point to the pendant hanging around her beautiful sister's neck.

For a split moment, the world and time stood still for both of them. All the wonderful memories they had together as sisters over the years came flooding back.

Mum smiled, and not only with her mouth. She smiled with her eyes. With her skin. Her smile came from her heart and soul. The love between them as sisters needed no words. Communication between them was now at the most profound level, through their hearts. Mum was unable to speak, but she knew, through the emerald crystal pendant, she was forever loved by her sister. It was a moment of pure joy. Mum then closed her eyes. She looked at peace.

In the last few days of Mum's life, she appeared to emotionally connect to one of the nurses in the hospice, called Mary. Mary was gentle, compassionate, and kind to Mum. She would sit and talk to Mum for ages and would not leave her side.

On that Saturday evening, Mary came in and was attending to Mum's morphine medication and making her comfortable in bed. Mary managed to sit Mum upright.

Mum suddenly held out her arm. She then grasped Mary's arm. Mary immediately leaned over the bed towards Mum. Looking at Mary straight in the eyes, Mum managed to open her mouth and said in a quiet, weak voice, "Sorry."

Even then, when Mum was facing death, she was apologising for her illness and the trouble she was causing Mary. It was another very touching and moving moment.

Saying goodbye

The last two days of Mum's life were traumatic, but filled with such imperturbable beauty at the same time.

On Sunday night, I decided to sleep in Mum's room right next to her. As I arrived at the hospice, one of the nurses told me it was a beautiful thing to do.

"She is waiting for you to be by her side. She won't go until you are there," the nurse said gently.

I then asked the nurse whether she will die peacefully.

"Yes," she replied.

Mum was lying there, still and peaceful. Her eyes were closed. Lying beside her, I cradled her in my arms. Then I slipped my hand into hers. Spontaneously, her hands moved. She held my hands tightly. She wouldn't let it go. Her grip was so strong. I suddenly broke down in a flood of tears. This time though, my pain and heartache were indescribable. Like a nail driven into a tree, the pain once again pierced through my heart and soul. I felt so alone and so empty. I was completely rendered helpless. Suddenly, a nurse walked in the room. It was like an angel arrived, just at the right moment. She wrapped her arms around me.

She comforted me. "She knows you are here," the nurse added reassuringly. *"She is asking your permission to let go. She wants to know that you will be alright. That is the greatest gift you can give her right now, knowing that you will be okay."*

So I leaned over and whispered in her ear, "I love you. You can let go. I will be fine, thank you for being my Mum."

The nurse assured me that she could hear me. I don't know if that was true. But I kept saying I loved her.

"By holding your hand, she is leaving you a legacy of love," the nurse commented.

Then Mum opened her eyes. Even though they were fluttering, glazed and looking right through me, they were glittering with love. They were beautiful.

Mum moved her pale thin face towards me. She so desperately tried to say a word, but she simply did not have the energy or strength.

"Don't worry, I know. I love you, Mum," I responded.

Her sheer vulnerability stripped everything away to reveal the love within her soul. I understood, for the very first time in my life, the core of what it is to be human. The ultimate truth of Mum's life was love. She then closed her eyes. She moved her hand towards me. Mum gripped my hand for about three hours. Clasping onto each other, my arm was aching.

I attempted to slip my hand away, but she wouldn't let it go. She grasped my hand even tighter. My touch and my presence were the only comfort I could give her at this moment.

I comforted her, saying that I will always be here. Suddenly, around midnight, Mum completely loosened her grip. In a matter of seconds, her arm relaxed. I laid her arms on her chest. Her breathing got shallower as the fluid mucilage of the secretion rattled in her windpipe.

"She is relieved. She knows that everything is safe now. She can let go," the nurse remarked quietly.

I knew instinctively that Mum was entering the final few hours of life. The final separation was now inevitable. Mum's body was transitioning.

From now on, communication between us would not be based on words, but on physical touch.

When the nurses came in the room, they started to change her. I subsequently left the room. When I came back, I saw a tear had formed in her right eye and rolled down her cheek. I wiped her face. I immediately called the doctor. She agreed that Mum looked in distress at being changed. The doctor apologised and assured me they would be more careful the next time when they changed her.

I made up my bed next to her. All night I was talking to her. Her breathing was becoming longer. The secretion noise from her body was getting louder. The nurse reassured me, however, that Mum was not in any pain.

The nurses came in three times during the night to keep a check on her medication and to change the morphine syringe driver.

I didn't sleep that night; I felt rough. I left Mum at about 8:30 am to go home. As I left the room, I knew Mum was now physically, emotionally, and spiritually ready to go. It was just a question of hours now.

Last day

On the last day of Mum's life, I drew upon and tested my faith as I never had done so before.

My faith allowed me to confront my own personal anguish

in such a way that gave me hope and allowed me to forgive. It was not going to protect me from the reality of life.

I was fortunate, as I had a mature understanding of death. I recounted to myself what Marcus Aurelius (who was the Roman Emperor from 161 AD to 180 AD) said:

"Pass then through this little space of time conformably to nature, and end thy journey in content, just as an olive falls off when it is ripe, blessing nature who produced it, and thanking the tree on which it grew.

For death is part of nature."

As I was sitting with Mum in silence, a nurse walked in the room and introduced a trainee nurse.

"Can you please remove the trainee nurse?" I contested angrily. "This is a private moment."

The nurse apologised.

As Mum's body was in the process of dying (at this stage she was in a comatose state), I asked for Paul, the hospice chaplain to enter the room. He was wonderful. He provided me with immeasurable solace and comfort. He prayed for Mum. Afterward, he said a prayer for me.

There were no tears, just tranquillity and peacefulness in the room. Silence does not lie. There was pure divine acceptance of Mum and her soul.

Mum's stillness was beautiful. As she first saw me take my first breaths entering this world, she allowed me the privilege and profound honour to witness taking her last breaths departing the world. Seeing Mum lying there, I knew that her natural death was nothing to be scared of. It was part of life.

As strange as it may sound, the precious few hours I spent with Mum, I can only describe as full of pure beauty. There we were, just Mum, Paul and myself in the room.

There was something deeply profound witnessing the sheer vulnerability of another human being, who happened to be my Mum. Through the purity of her love, I could feel the integrity of her soul. I knew her soul was leaving her body. I knew however, her soul would be very much alive in my heart. Through the silence and stillness, I felt a divine presence.

As her son, in my heart, I had to let her go. I needed to hand her over.

Through my love for her, I accepted, it was now her final journey to take alone. I was also aware of the consequences of not letting her go at that moment, as my heart might as well have stopped beating in the room too. I understood, however, it was her time to depart from the world, and not mine. I knew I had to keep on living.

Nevertheless, it felt like I lost half my heart that day. And even today, it still feels that way.

I repeated to Mum that I loved her and thanked her for giving me a wonderful life.

"Your mum is nearing the end," the nurse whispered to me. "She has only minutes to live."

I consciously decided not to be in the room when Mum took her final last breath. It was her time to take death's hand. That was between her and God only. I advised the nurse of my decision. She agreed it was a good decision.

"Your mum will not be awake when she takes her last breath," the nurse told me. "She will not recover from her unconscious state. She won't know she will be taking her last breath, it will just happen."

So I decided to wait in the waiting room to be told the news. But no one came round to see me.

Six o'clock came, seven o'clock passed, and Mum was still alive.

By 7:30 in the evening, I had a sudden thought in my mind. Every half hour, I would go into Mum's room, kiss her on the forehead, and say that I loved her.

So I did. Eight o'clock. Eight-thirty.

Then, at nine o'clock in the evening, as I went to walk into Mum's room, the nurse stopped me.

"Has she gone?" I asked.

"Yes," she replied.

The nurse then gently held my hand.

"Can I see her?" I asked.

"Yes," the nurse replied.

The nurse physically held onto me as I walked into the room.

Mum was still and motionless.

For the final time, I told her that I loved her, and I thanked her. I kissed her on the forehead for the very last time.

I experienced a peace and transcendent serenity that passed beyond my understanding. I knew that death would not separate us.

The woman who had brought me into the world looked at peace. I was comforted by the fact that I was there at the very end. Nevertheless, there was a suddenness about it. Mum's passing happened much more quickly than I expected. But what really struck me, was the finality of death. Mum's life was now over. I left Mum's room and walked back to the waiting room. The design of which was both beautiful and breathtaking. It had an elegant, contemporary feel to it. It was full of light due to its soaring glass ceiling and large window panels.

While it was just after 9 pm, it was still light outside. As I looked up to the ceiling, I saw a single tree. I could see the wind roaring through it as it swayed from side to side. Every leaf was battling to survive to stay on. For ten minutes, I just couldn't take my eyes off this particular tree. And then suddenly, the wind dropped, and the leaves were safe again.

Before I left the hospice, I went back to see Mum. The door was open. I stood outside the room as the nurses attended her. They were in the process of wrapping a towel around her head and jaw. I said goodbye to her and repeated the Lord's Prayer.

I was calm. I was not crying. I simply felt profoundly honoured. I have witnessed an event of pure beauty that even the words in this book cannot fully describe. And nor should they. There are certain times in life where meaning and words are simply inadequate. I felt something within my heart change.

As I slowly walked back to the waiting room, I called Mum's brothers and sisters. It was now pitch dark outside. I looked up to the glass ceiling again. The weather had suddenly changed. I could see a thunderstorm brewing.

I left the hospice at 11 pm. It was eerily quiet. As I walked out the door, a gust of wind blew into my face. It was now raining, windy, and cold. I felt Mum was with me as I walked home that evening.

As I arrived home, I went straight to bed.

I woke up in the middle of the night. It must have been around 3 am. I felt restless. I then started to play some songs on my iPad.

Somehow, for whatever reason, my Internet connection had crashed. Usually, I would just reset the connection. That evening, however, I was too exhausted to do even that. So I just decided to look for tracks that I could play without the connection.

But out of around 300 song tracks on my iPad, I could only play five songs.

Those five songs, however, were precisely what I needed that evening. They comforted, resonated, and spoke deeply to my heart and soul.

I am not going to reveal these songs, but merely ask you: what five songs would you have chosen if you were in my position that evening?

Before I fell asleep, reality hit me. I knew when I woke up the next morning Mum would not be there.

Next days

It was hard to explain how I felt when I woke up the next morning.

Knowing that I would never see her again, I felt shocked and numbed. I realised it was a new chapter in my life.

That morning I took a shower and had breakfast. Then my mind went into practical mode. I looked at my charter for one final time before I took it down off my bedroom wall. It had served its purpose. "Take one day at a time," I reminded myself.

I was aware nevertheless, I had to register Mum's death at the local register office. But first, I had to collect a form from the doctor in the hospice. That morning, I walked into the hospice. The nurses were so tender and caring towards me. I knew Mum was still in her room. It felt strange. I felt her spirit within me.

"Do you wish to see her?" a nurse asked tenderly.

"No. Thank you," I replied.

I knew deep within my heart that I had said my final goodbye to Mum the previous night.

To see her body again would not be right, and it would spoil the spirituality and preciousness of the moment last night.

I collected the certificate and immediately took a bus to the marriages and deaths registrar office in Kensington, London.

The registrar examined the document and advised that the certificate was incomplete.

While the time of Mum's death was recorded, the doctor at the hospice failed to record the last time she saw Mum alive.

I argued with him. He eventually rang the hospice. Thankfully he spoke to the relevant doctor and accepted the certificate.

The registrar then gave me the death certificate and a form (known as the Green Form) to take to the funeral directors.

Mum discussed her funeral wishes beforehand with me. She didn't mind what happened to her. She preferred cremation, simply because it was cheaper. "Don't spend too much money on me," she used to say to me.

Paul guided me on the best course of action to take. He persuaded me to cremate Mum and then at a later date, I could intern her ashes where her mother has been laid to rest.

I agreed to have a church service. There was something inside me that could not accept Mum being cremated. So once the church service was over, I decided that I would walk out and leave Mum in the church. Paul would then accompany Mum to the crematorium. Her ashes would be held by the Funeral Director, until such date, I felt emotionally stable to intern her ashes.

I received beautiful condolence and sympathy cards from family, friends, and neighbours. Their words were heartfelt and so comforting. So much so, I have kept them to this day. But at the time, I simply could not comprehend that the cards were for me. Why I am I receiving them? I have never received sympathy cards in my entire life. Surely there was some mistake. Seeing them lined up on the windowsill seemed so surreal. Then one afternoon, I crumbled to my knees as the reality hit me right between the eyes. It was then I fully understood—yes, Mum has died.

Funeral service

I agonised over the funeral service. I arranged the service on Tuesday, 16th June 2015. The Saturday before, I completely broke down and convinced myself I was not going to attend. I just couldn't handle it. But somehow, I pulled myself together. My eulogy was short and simple:

EULOGY – VERBATIM

I want to tell the world about my Mum.

Mum was an amazing and beautiful woman. Her needs were simple. Simple things in life made her happy. She never once thought of herself first. She was strong, resilient, and stoic.

Mum's heart was full of pure love. I was Mum's pride and joy. I was her world.

Caring for Mum over the past year was second nature. It was as natural as breathing. I was deeply honoured to walk beside you in your hour of darkness. I was privileged to see her beautiful soul and her beautiful spirit.

To me, her soul and spirit are as real as I see you. I can touch it. I can feel it. It is inside me now.

I wish to thank you for being my Mum. I could not ask for a better Mum. Your gentleness, your support, but most of all, I wish to thank you for always loving me.

I wished I had a few more years with you on Earth, but God decided to take you into his Kingdom now. Don't worry Mum, I have prayed to him, and he has told me that Heaven holds a special place for you.

I want you to know, you were born in love. You lived 80 years in love. And you have passed away in my love.

My grieving will never stop. More importantly, my love for you will never stop.

Whilst I am living, I will make you proud. I will make all of your sacrifices worth it. For everything, I thank you. You have given me an amazing life.

And your love, Mum, will always be inside me until the day I join you. END OF EULOGY.

I waited three months after the funeral before I interned Mum's ashes. I remember the day vividly; it was a nice and sunny day. I needed time to think on my own. My heart was crying out for solitude, silence, and peace. On that particular afternoon, I suddenly found myself, walking through a beautiful country lane. The air smelt of herbs. I was alone with no one in sight for miles. As I walked, I passed a row of trees. There were five trees on each side of me.

Then suddenly out of nowhere, an idyllic breeze blew up. I stopped and looked ahead.

Out of the five trees on my right-hand side, only one tree had its leaves blowing in the breeze. I stood there and simply took a deep breath. I could not believe what I was seeing.

I knew instinctively that was Mum. I knew she was with me and watching over me.

Hence the title of this book, *Peaceful Breeze*.

12

Grief is the price we pay for love

I believe grief of a loved one is one of the most painful experiences you will endure. For me, it pierced right through my heart. Love and grief go hand in hand, like night and day. You can't have one without the other.

You only need to turn on the television and watch the news where we see death thrust in our faces. But it does not dramatically affect us. That is because essentially grief is about either an emotional or physical connection that has been lost. In short, we do not grieve for people we do not know. Grief is therefore a response to what we have loved and cherished.

Many years ago, I remember a distinguished psychologist once commented on measuring grief. He highlighted a 'Grief Intensity Scale'. The scale started from zero to five (zero representing no emotion and five representing complete despair). I found this tool useful. For the first few weeks after Mum passed away, I wanted to understand my own approach to grief. Using this scale, I scored myself around four out of the possible five points. Now however, as the months have passed, I fluctuate around the score of two or three on the scale. I believe it will remain around that level for the rest of my life.

I am no expert on grief. Like everyone else, I continue to this day to stumble and flounder around like someone in a pitch-dark room, having no clue as to where to find the light switch.

But I soon gathered that there is no one size to grieving.

Or a right way or wrong way to grieve. Experiencing grief is different for everyone and, therefore, people cope with the loss of a loved one in their unique way. In my opinion, grief is an individual thing. No one can feel my pain, nor should they. No one can take the pain away from me. You can't simply switch off the pain of losing a loved one like a tap. At least, my grief didn't work like that.

Grief is usually complex. Well it was for me. I found it an isolating and lonely experience. The vast ocean of grief was ready and waiting to drown me. I consciously decided, however, not to sink to its depths in despair but to surf its waves. In short, I consciously embraced my grief rather than running away from it or denying it. This meant taking a risk. It meant allowing myself to lose control of all of my emotions and not to be scared, apologetic, embarrassed of breaking down. I accepted that I would be blown back and forward by all of my feelings. And so there I was, with a force greater than a storm in the middle of the Atlantic Ocean, looking grief straight in the eye.

At random moments during the day, I would just burst into tears. The pain in my heart would be, at times, crippling, like a knife had been stabbed not only through my heart but also through my soul. There are still occasions when I think, even today, she is still here. I am going to hear her voice again. She hasn't really died—no, not Mum. She is immortal. But of course, once again, reality hits me right through the eyes.

Personally, it would be the little and trivial things I would deeply and profoundly miss and find upsetting. It is at these times I would feel the pain and hurt more acutely. Making Mum a bacon sandwich on a Sunday morning. Making her a cup of tea. Boiling her an egg. They would all trigger profound and painful emotions inside of me. Never to hear her sweet and tender voice is heartbreaking. But by losing control and allowing myself to feel the rawness of my pain, day by day, I somehow got through the trauma.

The hobbies and pastimes I used to dearly love felt

insignificant. "What's the point of that?" I repeatedly asked myself.

I also yearned for Mum to come back to be with me. Every time I went out shopping, I would see Mum ahead of me, either in the street or down a supermarket aisle. I would run up to her with joy and relief. Even calling out her name. As I would move closer to her, she would turn round. Then time and time again, reality would hit me. Because, of course, it would always be a total stranger who I thought resembled Mum. They might have had the same type of overcoat on as Mum, the same style of grey hair as Mum, or simply had the same walking style as Mum. On every occasion, my heart would sink as the harsh reality dawned. I will never see Mum again in this life.

The well-publicised stages of grief introduced by Elisabeth Kübler-Ross in 1969 set out the emotional stages of grieving that are denial, anger, bargaining, depression, and acceptance, which were originally an observation of dying patients.

I am not going to criticise this grieving model as clearly it helps and comforts many thousands of people. The fact is, it simply did not help me in my personal grieving journey.

I naturally thought that grief was a linear step-by-step process and I would simply snap out of it. I could not be more wrong. My grief was at times chaotic and turbulent as I crawled in and out of my emotional abyss. Day after day, a whole raft of emotions, ranging from guilt, shame, sadness, anger, and emptiness would overlap in my mind. Sometimes, I would sway from one emotion to another in an hour, or even in a course of one minute.

The most dominant emotion that pervaded my mind, however, was one of guilt. Guilt, I believe, is one of the most difficult emotions to cope with because it follows you around. It pervades your mind. And so it was for me. Ruminating over and over again in my mind, was one key question. Could I have done more for Mum?

After a long, hard and painful journey, I found that it was

through forgiveness, I finally found peace within myself. Stillness of my heart was what pulled me through the grieving process.

Through my serenity, I acknowledged the concept of permanence, that is to say, everything in life is temporary, and that even includes, heartbreakingly, the people I love.

I, therefore, had two stark choices in front of me in life. Did I simply curl up in a ball and shut the world out and just survive day by day and wait until my time is up so I could meet Mum again? Or did I use the love in my heart that Mum has left me and live the best life I could?

And as strange as it may seem, I not only considered the former option, I genuinely felt at times I wanted just to give up on life, as part of me died when Mum passed away.

A good friend sent me a quote by a text message. It said: "When our actions are based on good intentions, our soul has no regrets." Therefore as much I tried, I could not deny the love within my heart. So no matter how much pain or grief pervaded my heart, it was love that has pulled me through. I realised at that very moment, what makes us truly human, when you strip everything away and become your authentic self, is love.

By allowing myself to feel my grief, the rawness of the pain within my heart, was softened. In time, memories of Mum have turned into beautiful roses brightening up the garden of my mind. That is not to say my heart is not broken. It is. It will never be the same. I miss Mum every single day. The best I can hope for is to learn to live with it. As Mum allowed me the privilege to see the purity of her soul, I honestly believe grief has taught me to be more humble than ever before, to be more compassionate than ever before, to be more grateful for what I have in life and to be kinder than ever before. In many ways, I'm a more joyful, soulful and humble person.

As mentioned, I am not an expert on grief. Whilst I am conscious not to provide you with advice, I would, however, like to highlight four things that worked for me. They may not work for everyone.

First, I understood that I had to let go. It was Mum's journey when she was passing away. I had a different journey to take, one of grieving and then living the best life possible. Talking was good, but ultimately, in the middle of the night, I was alone. Therefore, acknowledging and accepting was key in not allowing my life to be ripped apart by Mum's death.

Second, maintaining a sense of connection with Mum. By writing this book, for instance, I have started to integrate Mum into my present and future life. Mum is with me more than she has ever been. I also continue to follow my personal rituals that comfort me. These could be seen as silly and inconsequential to anyone looking in from the outside, but for me, they were and continue to be deeply meaningful. For example, I light a candle for Mum whenever I can. I talk to Mum on a daily basis. I know she can hear me.

Third, I was determined to be kind to myself. I believe self-compassion is key in dealing with my grief. In practical terms, this meant not being too hard on myself, not beating myself up about being sad and trying to understand my feelings more. I also allocated 'personal grief time' for myself each day. Putting aside time each day so I consciously remember Mum and the wonderful times we had together.

Finally, I never gave up on life. I continued to keep myself both mentally and physically active. Not only did I eventually continue with my hobbies, I proactively sought new things to do with my life that stretched my personal capability as well as giving me a sense of achievement and purpose.

Shakespeare once said about death that it was the undiscovered country from which no traveller returns. But is that really true?

No doubt social psychologists such as Freud, who had little regard for religion or spirituality, would fully endorse this sentiment by Shakespeare.

Since Mum passed away, I have now begun to see manifestations. These could be seeing white feathers intermittently around the house, which is unusual, as I never noticed them before Mum passed away.

Or a butterfly found in my bedroom. Or a gentle breeze on my face on a quiet, sunny day.

Is Mum trying to tell me she is okay? Are the feathers being left by an angel to reassure me that she is fine? Or am I, as Freud would argue, unconsciously looking for coincidences to comfort myself? Or even imagining the manifestations? The truth is – I simply do not know. You would, however, not be human if you did not yearn for someone you loved who passed away. It is a basic, fundamental human condition.

What I do know, however, is that whenever I find a white feather lying around the house, or a gentle breeze on my face, I feel contented, warm, and full of love.

I, therefore, have chosen to believe in something higher and greater than myself. There is in my opinion, something that continues after death. I believe Mum is communicating to me in different manifestations that now occur in my life. I know Mum is with me in the air, the wind, and is now part of Mother Nature. For me, her soul is not extinguished.

Final chapter

There are 330,000 patients diagnosed with cancer each year in the UK, which one in four present to doctors when it is too late. My Mum was one of those patients. While I was in the centre of the storm and my world was falling apart, I just could not understand or comprehend her thought processes of not going to see the doctor. Looking back, I can now appreciate Mum's rationale for refusing to see the doctor until, sadly it was too late.

Her logic was not linear or straightforward, but was multi-layered and full of emotion and was consistent with how she lived her life and who she was. I believe there were a number of reasons why she acted in this way: inertia, denial, being scared and, upon reflection, her immense embarrassment of being ill. Throughout her entire life, she did not want to trouble or be a burden to anyone and her illness was going to be no exception.

Through the act of acceptance and loving, I believe Mum had a good, calm, and peaceful death. As strange as it may sound, her passing was dignified and beautiful. She passed away naturally in God's time and was pain free.

I feel deeply honoured that I was able to be with Mum during her final moments.

I was witness to something I could never have imagined. I saw beyond the human body.

I felt a pure and transcended love, which was far beyond my comprehension and understanding and impossible to articulate in words.

She gave me the gift of showing me the purity and integrity of her eternal soul. This truly humbling experience has led me to believe that the human body and soul are separate.

The day Mum passed away, I realised that something had profoundly changed within me. It renewed my belief that death only occurs to the body. Death is the process of life. I believe Mum's body may have died, but her soul has simply moved on. I don't need physical proof, I know she is here with me.

Whenever I see the trees blowing in the wind or a soft breeze hits my face, I know she is saying something to me. I feel her guidance. She is still looking after me. And, as silly as it may seem, I talk back to the trees. I will continue to talk to the trees until my last breath.

I now know that Mum is in a better place. She is with her mum and her brothers.

The true testament to Mum is that she never, ever wanted to give up. She so much wanted to live. Even during the last few days of her life, she was still fighting.

I wondered how my faith would withstand the emotional turmoil and heartache of accepting Mum's terminal illness and then accepting her passing away. To my amazement, I discovered, it was precisely when I was facing the worst period of my life, to such an extent, that I doubted my faith, my faith grew and strengthened. Faith turned my darkness into light, my fear into love and my sadness into joy.

Faith is now integral to the way I live. It helps me to navigate the cruel seas of life. And believe me, nothing can be more cruel in life than seeing someone you love die in front of your very eyes and you are rendered completely powerless. It was my faith that steered me into a calm harbour where I returned to still waters of peace and tranquility.

Even though I cherished Mum when she was alive, it was not until her death, I realised what a truly remarkable woman she was. The old adage, you don't know what you have until its gone is so very true.

Throughout her life, there was one lesson above all else that

Mum taught me, namely of inner contentment and peace. I have now found comfort in the simple and mundane things in life. In short, I have found comfort in simply being me. It is an inner contentment that no one can take from me.

I am now less afraid of life than I was before. I am conscious of the fact of living life with abundance. The direction of my life has dramatically changed. I am following my passions like never before. I am determined to reinvest all my energies into the present and future. Mum would want to see me get out there and achieve what she believed I could do. Mum would have wanted one thing above all else for me, that is to be happy.

I believe, if you condense it down and strip everything away, life is really about love. We are put on this world to love and to be loved. The most important relationship we will ever have, however, is with ourselves.

As hard it is for me to say, Mum's physical body is now just dust. As life goes on, who is going to remember her in years to come? The simple answer – no one. She is now one of the anonymous dead. I know however, she graced her time on earth with kindness and love. For me, that is what being alive is about. Mum is not unique. Despite, today's harsh world, the majority of people on this earth, and certainly the people I meet in my life, are kind, loving and wonderful.

Death is not the end. I believe there is a connection beyond the physical form. My relationship with Mum is still alive within a deep inner space within my heart. Her strength lives in me. And will remain so until we reunite.

I have found one cliché or platitude that I have realised has been true for me. Life is about the journey and not about the destination. Both as a son and as a carer, I have been on an incredible journey. Every moment of the day, I have lived that journey. I am no different to the millions of carers in the world who have their own remarkable and inspirational stories to tell.

For my final words, I wish to leave you to contemplate the comforting lyrics of the life-affirming song by Rogers and Hammerstein from the film *Carousel*, *You Never Walk Alone*.

The lyrics gave me comfort when looking after Mum as they do now – living my life with confidence and with a purpose.

Mum, you will never walk alone.

Rest in Peace.

www.ingramcontent.com/pod-product-compliance
Lightning Source LLC
Chambersburg PA
CBHW031627040426
42452CB00007B/714